H & P:
A Nonphysician's Guide to the Medical History and Physical Examination

Third Edition

John H. Dirckx, M.D.

Health Professions Institute • Modesto, California • 2001

H & P: A Nonphysician's Guide
to the Medical History and Physical Examination
Third Edition

by John H. Dirckx, M.D.

Copyright © 2001 by Health Professions Institute

First Edition 1987; Second Edition, Revised, 1991
Published by Health Professions Institute

Cover design by Lori Raven Smith

Published by

Health Professions Institute
P. O. Box 801
Modesto, California 95353
Phone 209-551-2112
Fax 209-551-0404
Web site: http://www.hpisum.com
E-mail: hpi@hpisum.com

Sally Crenshaw Pitman, Editor & Publisher

Printed by
Parks Printing & Lithograph
Modesto, California

ISBN: 0-934385-34-3

Last digit is the print number: 9 8 7 6 5 4 3 2 1

For Joyce

Foreword

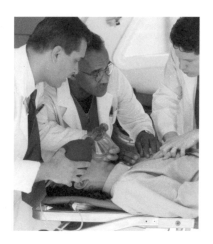

This book will not make a diagnostician of anyone. Its purpose is to acquaint nonphysicians with the nature and nomenclature of the medical history and physical examination as currently performed and recorded by physicians. Although directed principally to medical transcriptionists, it should also be helpful to medical secretaries, nurses, clinical psychologists, social workers, insurance clerks, lawyers, and other nonphysicians who are called upon to handle or interpret medical records.

The importance of the history and physical examination in medical practice can hardly be overstated. Medicine might be defined as an art and science whose goals are the prevention, identification, and treatment of human diseases, including the results of injury, developmental abnormalities, and degenerative and malignant processes. Some diagnosis, at least general or provisional, must precede any rational attempt at treatment. Since both a review of the patient's complaints and some kind of systematic examination are basic and indispensable elements in the diagnostic process, it would be hard to imagine an instance of medical treatment to which history and physical are wholly irrelevant. Moreover, history and physical examination are often performed when no disease is suspected and no treatment is contemplated, as in a routine health checkup or a preemployment physical.

Whether the history and physical are narrowly restricted to the area of a specific problem, such as a cut finger, or are performed on an elaborate and exhaustive scale, a permanent record must be preserved in writing in either printed or electronic form. The written report of a history and physical examination not only serves to supplement the memory of the treating physician but may also provide essential information to other physicians months, years, or decades later. In addition, it may assume great legal significance, documenting the thoroughness and appropriateness of the physician's evaluation and the accuracy of the diagnosis, providing a basis for health insurance benefit payments, or supplying data for disability determination or workers' compensation.

Medicine, like every other profession, has its own intricate and arcane idiom, some of it formal and recorded in dictionaries and textbooks, some informal, colloquial, and evanescent. Much of this latter kind of jargon pertains to the art of physical diagnosis and is used by physicians in recording historical details and physical findings. A considerable part of this jargon consists of formal terms used in unconventional ways. (For example, the phrase *no pathology in the pelvis* has nothing to do with either the formal subject matter of the science of pathology or the bones collectively termed the pelvis in anatomy.) Hence, even a person with a thorough understanding of basic medical terminology and access to medical dictionaries and reference works may find some clinical records misleading or unintelligible. The fact that the art of diagnosis has its own special brand of logic, not easily followed by persons who have never practiced medicine, adds further to the difficulties of the lay person who must transcribe medical records from dictation or peruse them in quest of information.

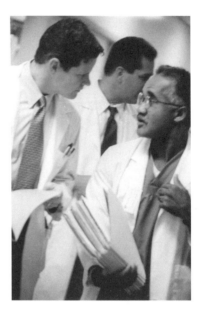

Several features combine to make this book a valuable resource for transcriptionists and other nonphysicians who deal with medical records. I have described each step of the history and physical examination in a separate chapter. Excerpts from a variety of H&P reports appear in shaded boxes immediately following the text to which they refer. In addition, for reference and comparison, relevant words and phrases appear in side bars labeled "For Quick Reference." Throughout the book, medical jargon is discussed and defined on an equal footing with formal terminology. Words and phrases not found in standard references are defined in a glossary at the end of the book.

If medical transcriptionists and health information management personnel find this book helpful, let them take it as a small return for the unpayable debt that physicians and their patients owe these unsung and generally invisible but diligent and indispensable members of the healthcare team.

About the Exercises

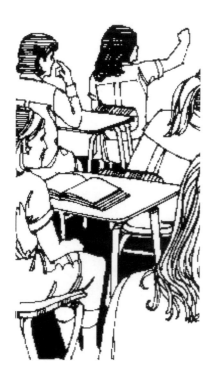

This third edition of *H&P: A Nonphysician's Guide to the Medical History and Physical Examination* has been expanded to include a variety of exercises contributed by educators. At the end of each chapter are multiple choice, fill in the blank, and short answer questions. There are also learning activities designed for individuals as well as small and large groups. As a study technique, it is a good idea to review the exercises at the end of each chapter before reading the chapter. If you are an independent study student, don't ignore the group activities; you may be able to adapt some of them to your situation. See the note to independent study students below.

The following headings are a guide to the kinds of questions and activities included:

Review and Summarize
Pause and Reflect
Relate and Remember
Collaborate and Share
Explain and Learn
Relax and Play
Generalize and Apply
Compare and Contrast
Extrapolate and Project

Some activities will require "going outside the text" for more information. Others will draw on your knowledge of anatomy, medical terminology, and disease processes. If you have not yet studied these topics, or are studying them concurrently with this text, you may have a little extra work to do. None of the activities, however, require that you be proficient in medicine in general or any specialties in particular. Since many of the activities involve collaboration with classmates, it is likely that your combined knowledge and experiences will suffice.

The exercises in this book may at first appear redundant, but there is a reason for this. Every attempt has been made to address different learning styles; thus, multiple choice, fill in the blank, and short answer questions may all seem to relate to the same general topic or point. Both the repetition and the different approaches to the same information help you to remember important points. Activities may be similar as well. Group activities may build on activities designed for individual students. Time and environment may limit completing all activities; it is not expected that an instructor require students to complete every question and activity at the end of every chapter.

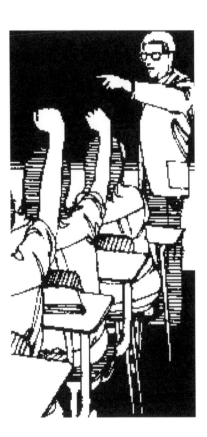

A Special Note to All Students. The questions and activities in this book have been designed to appeal to a variety of learning styles, one of which will work best for you. However, no single method of learning will work well for any individual all the time, and no single method of learning is suited to all material to be learned. All students use multiple learning styles to evaluate, digest, and incorporate new information into their experience and make it their own. For most, however, one style will predominate and be more comfortable than others. You are encouraged to stretch yourself beyond your comfort zone and attempt to answer all questions in these exercises, regardless of their form, and to participate in all the activities assigned by your instructor. In that way, you will ensure maximum retention and understanding of the material you are studying. A side benefit will be that you will teach yourself new learning techniques that will improve your performance in all your areas of study and enhance lifelong learning.

Note to Independent Study Students. Many of the group activities are easily modified to allow completion by an individual working alone. If multiple parts of an activity are divided among several students, complete all the tasks yourself. If you are to discuss or explain your findings to another person or to the group, write your explanation in a journal. You will be able to use this journal later as a study aid. For role-play activities or games, involve friends or family members. If you have Internet access, you can locate other independent study students at a networking Web site for medical transcriptionists and invite them to participate in on-line versions of group activities.

Note to Instructors. Answers to objective questions are included in the back of the textbook. Some of the questions and many of the activities are more open-ended and more subjective. For some of these, some guiding criteria are included. Others are purely subjective and there is no "right" answer. Many of the activities involve bringing in supplies (plain brown paper bags, sheets of butcher paper, colored pencils or crayons, colored dots or stars). When you assign a chapter to be read, you may want to assign the questions for the individual student as homework and plan for the group activities for the next class

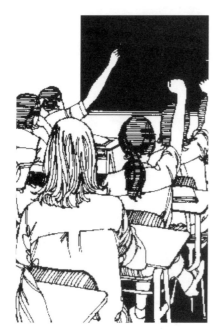

meeting. You can have the students themselves bring in any necessary supplies, or you may want to start the term with these supplies on hand in the classroom.

You are encouraged *not* to skip over the more participatory activities. Educational research has shown that these types of activities are the most successful for many if not most learners. In general, the activities included under the headings "Generalize and Apply" and "Extrapolate and Project" will be more difficult but will also be a sure gauge to whether (and how much) the students are actually incorporating the material into their experiences and fund of knowledge.

For the group activities, students should be encouraged to change groups and work with different students rather than always being in the same group with the same three or four people. Have students draw their group number from a box or bag. If you have five groups of five students, for example, write number 1 on five small pieces of paper, then 2, 3, and so on, up to 5. Mix the pieces up in a bag and let the students draw. The number they draw is the number of the group.

Another way to sort the students into groups is to use playing cards. Use the Ace, King, Queen, Jack, and 10 from multiple decks, five decks for five groups. Shuffle all the cards together and let the students draw a card. All the Aces become one group, the Kings another group, etc. Similarly, if you wanted only four groups, you could use one deck containing only the number of students you have in class and equal numbers of each suit. Then, all the hearts would go in one group, clubs in another, or use colored pieces of paper or similar objects (like paper clips, pencils, rubber bands, erasers) all placed into a bag from which each student draws or object. Like colors or like objects form a group.

Students, and you, may feel awkward and uncomfortable when first carrying out some of these activities, but soon they will be an important part of your classroom routine and all of you will look forward to them.

Health Professions Institute
Ellen Drake, CMT
Georgia Green, CMT
Linda Campbell, CMT

Art Acknowledgments

Photographic art used as illustrations in this edition was obtained from the *Medical Perspectives* and *Medicine & Health Care* series, available from EyeWire Images, Inc., www.eyewire.com.

Anatomical images were used with permission from *Super Anatomy Collection, LifeART Collections* (Baltimore: Lippincott Williams & Wilkins, 1995).

Labeled anatomical art was used with permission of Prentice Hall Health. The art was extracted from Health Professions Institute, *Medical Transcription Fundamentals & Practice*, 2nd ed. (Saddle River, NJ: Prentice Hall Health, 2000), from art originally appearing in Carole Miehl and Teresa England, *From Nursing Assistant to Clinical Care Associate* (Upper Saddle River, NJ: Brady Prentice Hall, 1999), and Francie Wolgin, *Being a Nursing Assistant* (Upper Saddle River, NJ: Prentice Hall Health, 2000).

Contents

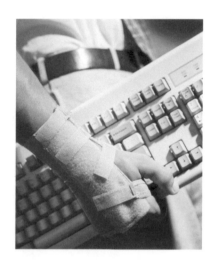

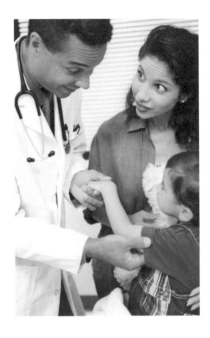

Introduction

General Principles of Physical Diagnosis

The term *diagnosis* (from Greek *diagignosko* "to judge, discriminate") has several closely related meanings in medicine, which few of us take the trouble to distinguish in practice.

Diagnosis means, first, the intellectual process of analyzing, identifying, or explaining a disease. In this sense, diagnosis forms the subject matter of the branch of medicine called Physical Diagnosis.

Secondly, in a somewhat more concrete sense, diagnosis means the explanation proposed for a given patient's problems. Thus we speak of "arriving at a diagnosis" or of "making a tentative diagnosis of pancreatitis."

Thirdly, diagnosis is often used synonymously with disease or the name of a particular disease: "Her diagnosis is multiple sclerosis." "Patients with this diagnosis often progress to renal failure."

Although we often talk about diseases as if they were real entities, disease is only an abstraction having no existence outside the mind. The notion of disease is a unifying concept by which we attempt to explain the origins and interrelations of a sick person's complaints and malfunctions. Physicians have adopted such concepts for the purely utilitarian purpose of simplifying and streamlining their thinking and talking about illness.

As the French physician and philosopher Alexis Carrel wrote more than 60 years ago in his book *Man, the Unknown*: "Disease is a personal event. It resides in the individual. There are as many different diseases as there are sick people. However, it would have been impossible to construct a science of medicine merely by assembling vast numbers of individual observations. The data had to be generalized and classified by means of abstractions. Those abstractions we call diseases."

Of course, the concept of specific diseases is not pure make-believe. There are more than enough similarities among cases of appendicitis, hepatitis C, or myocardial infarction to justify the use of these diagnostic categories and disease names. And yet, any candid observer must concede that our present system of nosology ("the classification of diseases," from Greek *nosos* "disease") embodies many grave flaws and inconsistencies.

Thus, we name some conditions according to their causes (*amebiasis, asbestosis*), others according to anatomic site (*conjunctivitis, pharyngitis*) or pathologic features (*cystic fibrosis, benign prostatic hyperplasia*), still others with purely descriptive epithets (*mallet finger, scarlet fever*). We preserve and

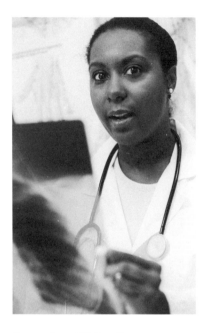

Learning Objectives

After careful study of this chapter, you should be able to:

Differentiate between *diagnosis* and *disease*.

Identify naming conventions for conditions.

Describe the process by which a medical diagnostician arrives at a diagnosis.

Identify variables that determine the extent and content of the history and physical exam.

Explain the significance of negative and positive findings.

Characterize the language of the report of the history and physical exam.

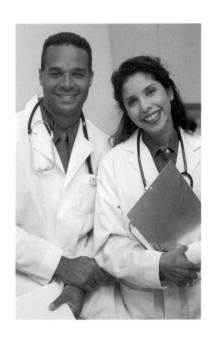

adapt terms from classical and medieval medicine (*cholera, influenza*) and even attach personal and place names to diseases (*Hashimoto thyroiditis, Lyme arthritis*). We use abstractions (*ulceration, telangiectasia*) alongside concrete terms (*peptic ulcer, sebaceous cyst*), even interchanging them at times, as when *cholelithiasis* becomes synonymous with *gallstones*. We make no linguistic distinction between highly specific terms (*toxoplasmosis*) and vague generic ones (*thyrotoxicosis*) or between diseases whose natures are well understood (*coronary arteriosclerosis*) and mere symptom complexes (*chronic fatigue syndrome*).

Most of these faults in classification and naming arise from peculiarities in the phenomena of disease, from gaps in our knowledge, and from limitations of language itself and the difficulty of altering a system of terminology that is codified in thousands of books and used daily by hundreds of thousands of professional people. With all their shortcomings, our current systems of classifying and naming diseases at least have the pragmatic justification that they "work"—in medical education, in the compilation of records and statistics, and in clinical practice.

Few physicians are logicians, much less philosophers. The "logic" of physical diagnosis is a rough-and-ready deductive process learned largely through imitation and experience. Its goal is the formulation of a diagnosis that will enable the physician to get on with the business of instituting rational treatment. Although founded on physics, chemistry, and other disciplines with rigidly mathematical bases, medicine is not and never can be an exact science.

The method of the medical diagnostician is an empirical one based upon a few elementary techniques and a "memory bank" of diseases and symptoms. A medical student learns not only the characteristic features of hundreds of diseases but also possible causes for each of hundreds of symptoms. Combining these two bodies of information—one, so to speak, vertical and the other horizontal—makes it possible to determine the most likely cause or causes for a given set of complaints or abnormalities. Starting with a specific problem—chest pain, fever, loss of appetite, inability to urinate—the physician considers the full range of diagnostic possibilities (called, in professional parlance, the "differential diagnosis," or simply the "differential") raised by that problem. Often the range is narrowed or modified from the outset by the patient's age, sex, or other readily evident factors. The physician tries to narrow the range of possibilities further and further by assembling more and more data until only one possibility remains.

The analytic process is actually far more complex than this simplified description of it would suggest. It involves establishing an accurate chronology of symptoms and events prior to the time the patient sought treatment, working out cause-and-effect relationships, and excluding irrelevant data ("red herrings") from consideration. In pursuing the ramifications of each new piece of information, the physician may adopt and reject ten or more working hypotheses in the course of two or three minutes.

Frequently, treatment of life-threatening problems such as cardiac or respiratory arrest or shock must accompany or even precede diagnostic evaluation. All too often, an exact diagnostic formulation remains impossible despite the most intensive investigation. When a patient is admitted to a hospital for diagnostic evaluation, the admitting diagnosis will necessarily be tentative or provisional, as reflected in such language as "Gastroenteritis, rule out early appendicitis, rule out pelvic inflammatory disease, rule out mittelschmerz."

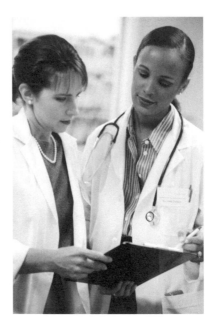

Although the collection and processing of diagnostic information eventually become second-nature for the physician, these activities never proceed with the mechanical rigidity and predictability of computer operations. Being human, physicians are subject to various forms of bias and error. They forget things, misinterpret what they see and hear, make mistakes of judgment, and may assign too much or too little weight to a given piece of information. On the other hand, with experience a physician acquires the ability to recognize and identify patterns—complex assemblages of historical and observed facts—in what seems to be a single, intuitive act of the mind. Such mental shortcuts can greatly simplify diagnosis but unfortunately they often yield wrong answers.

Such, then, is the intellectual basis of the diagnostic process. The techniques used by the physician to gather data for a diagnosis are embodied in the two procedures known traditionally as the history and physical examination. The history or anamnesis is an account of the subjective experiences—the *symptoms*—that constitute this episode of illness, as perceived by the patient and elicited by the diagnostician's careful, methodical questioning. Physical examination is the process whereby the physician seeks and observes objective changes and abnormalities—the *signs* of illness. It is not generally appreciated by lay persons that in a typical case, a skillfully obtained history supplies both a larger number of diagnostic clues and more useful and specific ones than the physical examination.

By convention, the term *physical examination* includes only those procedures performed directly by the physician relying on the five senses, with the aid of a few simple, handheld instruments. Although x-ray and laboratory studies, electrocardiography and electromyography, various kinds of scans, or other elaborate techniques may be absolutely essential to a precise and accurate diagnosis, they are not considered part of the physical examination.

The scope and nature of the history and physical depend on several variables. The patient's complaints give direction and focus to both history-taking and examination. The physician's field of specialization often determines the type and extent of diagnostic maneuvers employed. The setting of the examination—doctor's office or clinic, hospital emergency room, intensive care unit, or the patient's home—will have a bearing on what is done and not done. The patient's condition—whether alert, confused, belligerent, or unconscious—will influence the type of history that can be obtained and the degree of cooperation that can be enlisted during examination. Much may depend on formally established, quasi-legal requirements—forms to be filled out for a prospective employer or insurer or hospital staff bylaws to be complied with.

Our chief concern in this book is not the way the history and physical examination are performed but the way they are **recorded**. If we disregard all the variations that can possibly occur and take as an average or norm the type of history and physical examination generally performed on an adult patient

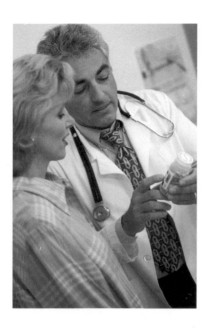

admitted to a hospital for the treatment of an acute illness or for an elective surgical procedure, we can identify some important recurring features of the written or dictated history and physical.

Usually there is some overlapping of content between the history and the physical examination. The physician does not wait until the history is completed to start observing the patient, nor do the questions stop once the examination starts. Hence the history may include a statement such as, "For about six weeks she has had a diffuse, nontender, nonfluctuant swelling on the dorsum of the left hand between the fourth and fifth metacarpals," where it is evident that some of the information has been supplied by the physician's own observation of the lesion.

A physical examination report might include the statement, "The abdomen shows a 7 cm transverse scar over the left costal margin due to a knife wound in childhood which apparently did not penetrate the abdominal cavity." The description of the scar is based on the physician's observations, but the explanation of its origin is obviously based on information provided by the patient. This information was probably not obtained while the history was being taken because the patient didn't think to mention it and the physician's questioning on the subject of prior injuries was not sufficiently searching to bring it out. Having learned about the lesion before actually dictating the history, the physician might have included it there, but in fact did not.

The report of a thorough history and physical contains more negative than positive statements: "He has had a mild chronic cough for many years but denies hemoptysis, purulent sputum, chest pain, dyspnea on exertion, orthopnea, asthma, bronchitis, or emphysema." This is because the physician is not concerned merely with compiling a list of abnormalities. A complete picture of the patient's condition must also indicate which common or relevant symptoms and signs are not present. Ordinarily it does not suffice to record simply that "there are no other complaints" or "the rest of the examination is negative." For several reasons, among them intellectual self-discipline and the need to document the thoroughness of the diagnostic process, the physician will usually record all "no" answers elicited in the course of history-taking and all normal findings in the physical examination.

The report of a history and physical as written or dictated by a physician is seldom a purely objective and descriptive document. In virtually every line one can discern the effects of interpretation, generalization, and inference. Perhaps we read, "The patient reports three-pillow orthopnea." Actually the patient said something like, "When I lie flat I feel like I'm smothering. I have to pile up about three pillows under my shoulders to get a decent night's sleep." The physician has translated this fragment of history into a familiar formula. Again, we may read that the patient has "a typical varicella rash." Instead of describing the rash, the physician has leapt at once to the diagnosis.

The language in which a physician writes or dictates a history and physical contains many recurring terms, phrases, and formulas. Some of these pertain to formal medical terminology, while others are highly informal, perhaps regional, institutional, or even individual, and do not appear in conventional medical reference works. An important characteristic of this language is its rigid economy, its tendency to abbreviate and condense wherever possible. It should be remembered that even a physician who dictates many pages of medical records a day may well produce at least as many pages of longhand in hospital charts and office or clinic records. Hence written abbreviations crop up constantly in dictated material, as when the physician dictates, "a mass in the subQ" for "a mass in the subcutaneous tissue," or "nocturia times three" (which would appear as "nocturia x 3" in a longhand note), meaning that the patient gets up three times a night to urinate.

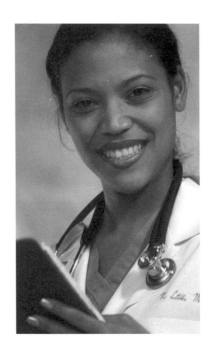

Compression of ideas and omission of connectives and even of whole phrases yield a terse and seemingly incoherent style of prose: "The heart is regular at 82 without murmurs, clicks, or rubs." "The face is symmetrical and the tongue protrudes in the midline." The physician who passes abruptly from a description of a painful, red, light-sensitive eye to the remark that the patient gives no history of pain or swelling in joints has not slipped a mental cog. The dictation has merely omitted a connecting phrase rendered unnecessary here by the fact that any other physician reading these remarks will know that arthritis occurs in several syndromes along with iritis (the tentative diagnosis in this patient).

Adding to the abstruseness of the workaday language of physicians is its heavy use of long, arcane, abstract words. This is not the place to explore the reasons why physicians feel compelled to say "experienced epistaxis" instead of "had a nosebleed," but the fact must be recognized that, in clinical records, technical words and phrases often replace simpler and plainer forms of expression. As in nonmedical settings, the grammar of dictated material tends to be exceedingly loose, with many incomplete sentences and syntactic breaks. The extent to which a transcriptionist amends and refurbishes what is dictated will depend in part on local conventions and institutional guidelines.

A few words about the format of this book. I have discussed the history and physical examination (H&P) step by step according to the following typical standard outline:

History
    Chief Complaint (CC)
        History of Present Illness (HPI)
        Family History (FH)
        Social History (SH)
        Habits
        Past Medical History (PMH)
            General
                Review of Systems (ROS)
                    Head, Eyes, Ears, Nose, Throat, Mouth, Teeth (HEENT)
                    Cardiovascular (CV)
                    Respiratory
                    Gastrointestinal (GI)
                    Genitourinary (GU)
                    Neuromuscular

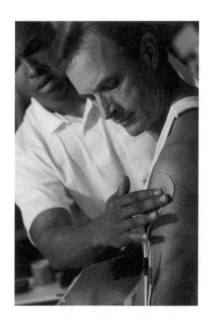

Review of Systems (ROS) *(continued)*
Psychiatric
Skin
Physical Examination (PE)
General Appearance
Skin
Head, Face, Neck
Eyes
Ears
Nose, Mouth, Throat, Teeth
Thorax, Breasts, Axillae
Heart
Lungs
Abdomen, Groins, Rectum, Anus, Genitalia
Back and Extremities
Neurologic
Formal Mental Status (Psychiatric)

Excerpts from H&P reports (including sentences and key words and phrases) appear throughout the text in shaded boxes, and in addition key words and phrases are listed alphabetically in For Quick Reference boxes as sidebars. The principal reason for this arrangement is to help the medical transcriptionist to decipher unclear passages of dictation. Italicized words and phrases in the shaded boxes are defined in the Glossary at the end of the book.

This book presupposes considerable knowledge of anatomy, physiology, and medical terminology, and access to standard reference works. Hence it neither defines *condyloma acuminatum* nor gives its correct plural. Nor does it purport to decide questions of usage (*Down's syndrome* vs. *Down syndrome*; *this data* vs. *these data*).

The Glossary is intended mainly to help with unusual words, unusual senses of common words, and jargon, including lay terms for diseases and symptoms that are not part of general English. Glossary definitions aim at brief accuracy rather than exhaustive precision.

Exercises for Introduction

Review and Summarize

A. Multiple Choice

Write the letter of the correct answer in the blank space before each multiple-choice question.

___ 1. Which of the following does NOT apply to disease?
   a. Diseases are named according to their cause.
   b. Diseases are named according to anatomic site or pathologic features.
   c. Disease is a concrete, distinct, easily identifiable entity.
   d. Disease is an attempt to explain the origins and manifestations of an illness.
   e. Disease is a personal event.

___ 2. Differential diagnosis is defined as
   a. The classification of diseases.
   b. The full range of diagnostic possibilities.
   c. An abstraction having no existence outside the mind.
   d. An account of the symptoms of an illness.
   e. A complete picture of the patient's condition.

___ 3. Which of the following is NOT normally part of the patient's history?
   a. A description of the onset and evolution of symptoms.
   b. A listing of possible symptoms the patient has not had.
   c. The recording of previous illnesses and surgeries.
   d. A description of the physician's observations of the patient.
   e. A discussion of the health of the patient's close relatives.

___ 4. The scope and nature of the history and physical depend on all of the following EXCEPT
   a. The physician's specialized field of medicine.
   b. The number of diagnostic procedures (x-rays, laboratory studies, EKG) performed.
   c. Whether the examination is in a doctor's office, clinic, ER, ICU, or patient's home.
   d. The patient's ability to answer questions and cooperate with the examiner.
   e. Formally established quasi-legal requirements.

B. Fill in the Blank

1. Disease is only a(n) _____ having no existence outside the mind.

2. _____ is a word meaning classification of diseases.

3. The admitting diagnosis is necessarily tentative or _____.

4. An account of the subjective experiences, or symptoms, of a patient is called a history or _____.

5. The process whereby the physician seeks and observes objective changes and abnormalities, generally using only the five senses and a few simple instruments, is called the _____.

C. Short Answer

Write a short definition of the following terms. If you can, condense the definition into just a few words or a single synonym that you feel more comfortable with. Find these words in the text. Do your synonyms make the narrative more clear? Note that the words are not always medical terms. Their application to the medical context may be different from their use in other contexts and may take some extrapolation on your part.

1. Subjective _____

2. Objective _____

3. Pathologic features _____

4. Epithets _____

5. Empirical _____

6. Inference _____

7. "Red herring" _____

8. Abstruseness_____

9. Arcane _____

10. Write 5-10 sentences summarizing five key points made in the introduction. Hints: importance of the history in arriving at a diagnosis, importance of the physical, two things you might have learned about disease, importance of positives and negatives, something about the language a physician uses in reporting findings.

_____

_____

_____

_____

_____

_____

Pause and Reflect

Think about your own experiences as a patient. If you have been fortunate enough never to have been a patient, consider the experiences of a relative or friend. You may even want to interview someone who has had extensive experience as a patient. Ask yourself or them questions such as these:

1. Describe the experience of visiting a doctor from the moment you were called from the waiting room until you left the examining room.

_____

_____

_____

_____

2. What kinds of questions were you asked? Who (nurse, physician, physician's assistant) asked them?

_____

_____

3. What procedures (weight, height, blood pressure, temperature, etc.) were performed? Who performed them?

_____

4. How extensive was the physical examination?

_____

5. What was the overall outcome of the visit? Were you given a diagnosis, prescription, referred to another doctor?

_____

_____

6. How much time did the entire visit take? How long were you with the physician? (The average patient-physician time during an office visit is 6 minutes.) What was your overall impression of the experience? How did you feel when it was over?

_____

_____

_____

As you read this text and complete the associated exercises, keep in mind your experience as described above.

Collaborate and Share

For the following activities, divide students into groups of 3 to 5. If possible, the groups should change for each activity.

1. Using your list of words from the Short Answer exercise above, discuss the statements in which these words are contained with others in your group until you all can explain what each statement means to the others.

2. Share your answers to Short Answer #10 above with the others in your group. As a group, condense all your responses into one response. Designate a representative to share your group's summary with the class.

Explain and Learn

1. In five or fewer sentences, explain the statement: Disease is only an abstraction having no existence outside the mind.

2. Is it the history or the physical examination that is more important in arriving at a diagnosis? Why?

Compare and Contrast

In light of the definition of *disease* above, discuss with your group how one disease is distinguished from another. Use specific diseases to illustrate your answers. You may use diseases familiar to the group members or compare and contrast diseases from a list supplied by your instructor or from the following: rheumatoid arthritis and osteoarthritis; upper respiratory tract infection (a cold) and influenza; gallbladder disease and appendicitis; pancreatitis and hepatitis.

Extrapolate and Project

1. Medical students learn the characteristic features (symptoms or findings) of hundreds of diseases, to which the term *vertical* is applied. They also learn the possible causes (trauma, pathogenic infection, environmental exposure, nutritional causes, aging, and so on), to which the term *horizontal* is applied. These two bodies of information make it possible for medical students to determine the likely cause(s) for a given set of complaints of abnormalities. Devise a chart or graph that might be used to compile these two bodies of information (one horizontal, one vertical) for either a single disease entity or a number of diseases, causes, and symptoms. For example, you might use a spreadsheet design listing different diseases vertically down the left margin. Horizontally, across the top, label columns with the causes listed above. Fill in an appropriate symptom for each disease in the column that corresponds to its cause. Relating disease/symptoms/causes in this way will help you to see relationships not only between these three parameters of an illness but relationships between different diseases sharing similar symptoms or causes.

2. Scan rapidly through the rest of the text. Can you hazard a guess as to how the study of this text might help you become a good transcriptionist? Try to state at least two things you see just by scanning that might improve your abilities as a medical transcriptionist or other allied health professional.

_____

_____

_____

_____

1

General Remarks on the History

As a rule, the physician compiles the medical history by questioning the patient. At times, however, much or all of the information must be obtained from someone else; considerable historical material may be drawn from written records. With experience, a physician learns to word questions so that they can be understood by a person of average intelligence, do not give offense or provoke hostility, elicit a maximum amount of relevant information with a minimum expenditure of time and effort, and do not suggest or invite specific answers. (A question like "You haven't had any sexual problems, have you?" virtually demands a negative reply.) Often the patient's response to one question determines what will be asked next, or how it will be asked. Little by little, a tolerably complete understanding of the patient's medical status, *as perceived by the patient*, emerges.

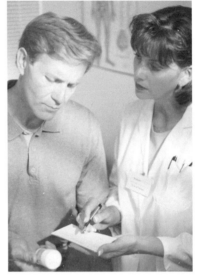

patient, examinee, subject, client
according to the patient's wife, husband, spouse, mother, father, parent, guardian
history obtained from the patient's girlfriend, boyfriend, companion,
    significant other
according to old records, hospital *charts*
history obtained with the patient's daughter acting as an interpreter

The volume and validity of information obtained through history-taking are limited by the informant's memory, intelligence, and ability and willingness to communicate. Anxiety provoked by being sick and having to see a doctor can severely hamper intellectual functioning. Even very bright lay persons usually lack extensive knowledge of human anatomy, physiology, and pathology, and so may have difficulty describing their problems clearly. Those who are not so bright or who are mentally ill have even more trouble. Memories are notoriously fallacious when it comes to recalling the dates of prior illnesses or operations, or even identifying them correctly.

Often the problem is too much information rather than too little. Some persons cannot keep to one subject but chatter on and on about irrelevant matters. If a patient seems particularly vague or unreliable in responding to an examiner's questions, the examiner may precede the recording of the history with a statement that this patient is a "poor historian"—partly to avoid the imputation of

Learning Objectives

After careful study of this chapter, you should be able to:

List the three primary sources for historical information.

Identify factors that limit the volume and validity of information obtained through history-taking.

Define the phrase *poor historian*.

Explain why a skilled and tactful interviewer seldom gets a fully unbiased and accurate history.

Identify factors that contribute to obtaining a good medical history.

Translate lay statements into medical jargon.

Propose a format for organizing random historical information.

For Quick Reference

gives a history of, relates, reports, states

believes, remembers, recalls

claims, insists, alleges

declines, refuses to discuss

only limited history is available, obtainable

anxious, apprehensive, distressed, disturbed, in acute distress, tense, upset

confused, inarticulate, incoherent, vague

noncommittal, reserved, reticent, taciturn, uncommunicative

cagey, evasive, hedging

candid, frank, open

hard of hearing, deaf

aphasic, mute

blasé, querulous, withdrawn

of limited, low, poor, substandard **intelligence**

diffuse, rambling, *tangential*   *logorrhea*

poor, unreliable, vague **historian**

articulates, *ventilates, verbalizes*

expresses, voices   multiple, numerous unrelated complaints

carelessness or ineptness if it should later appear that the history as recorded is grossly inaccurate.

Lay persons frequently misunderstand and distort technical terms and drug names, thinking, for example, that *hypertension* means excessive nervous tension, and saying "stationary tube" instead of "eustachian tube." Folk medicine, an ill-defined body of largely erroneous medical lore passed on from generation to generation among the laity, sometimes exerts a powerful influence on one's notions and even perceptions of one's own illness. A lay person (or, for that matter, a physician) may have false but unshakable convictions about the origin, nature, or proper treatment of an illness which color everything said about it to an interviewer. For these and other reasons, obtaining a good medical history demands alertness, flexibility, patience, the ability to appraise the patient's personality and emotional state quickly and accurately, and a great deal of finesse that can be acquired only through experience.

Few of us are entirely honest about our personal histories and habits, even when we know that the information may be important to our future health and well-being. We tend to filter out parts of the history that we don't want to reveal or discuss, and to distort the rest so as to fill in the blanks thus created. Although physicians rarely chide or ridicule patients and invariably respect their confidence unless medical or legal considerations force them to do otherwise, a patient may refuse adamantly to divulge information about sensitive issues such as family background, sexual behavior, or dietary practices. Again, we often think we can divine the bearing of an interviewer's questions and give answers that, though not literally true, supply the information we believe is needed or expected. Hence, even the most skilled and tactful interviewer seldom gets a fully unbiased and accurate history, even from an apparently candid and cooperative patient. When the whole of the history is a fabrication—as it sometimes is when the subject is psychotic, a malingerer, or a drug addict seeking to obtain a supply of some favorite poison through legitimate channels—the examiner's astuteness and diagnostic skill may be taxed to the utmost.

deceptive, mendacious	inconsistent, self-contradictory

The scope of the medical history depends on the reason for obtaining it, the patient's condition and ability to communicate, and many other factors. The following is a fairly standard format, though the order of the sections may vary somewhat.

Chief Complaint
History of Present Illness
Family History
Social History
Habits
Past Medical History
    General
    Review of Systems
        Head, Eyes, Ears, Nose, Throat, Mouth, Teeth
        Cardiovascular
        Respiratory
        Gastrointestinal
        Genitourinary
        Neuromuscular
        Psychiatric
        Skin

It must be emphasized that, although some such format is almost always followed in recording the patient's history, the information may have been obtained in much different order, perhaps even on more than one occasion or from a variety of sources. The answer to a dozen questions may be compressed into a single telling phrase. As mentioned earlier, the physician often translates the patient's statements into medical jargon. Thus, "I threw up at least five times" becomes, "He experienced emesis times five." On the other hand, the physician may make a point of quoting the patient's words exactly ("It feels like my intestines are all tangled around my heart.") or may fall into a colloquial style of dictation, unconsciously echoing the language actually used in interviewing the patient ("Since then he has had no more bellyache and is eating fine.").

In building up a complete picture of any given symptom, the physician asks a number of fairly standard questions. For example, with respect to pain—probably the commonest and most general presenting symptom—the physician inquires as to its quality, intensity, onset, duration, intermittency, location, and radiation, as well as any aggravating or alleviating factors, prior episodes of similar pain, and associated symptoms. The way in which this information is assembled can be seen in the following fictitious interview between a physician at a neighborhood clinic and a 54-year-old toolmaker with chest pain.

For Quick Reference

dead feeling
deaf
declines to discuss
deep in the joint
delimited
developed
diagnostic skill
diaphoresis
diarrhea
dietary practices
diffuse
dimensions
discomfort
distress, distressed
disturbed
divulge information
doubled up with pain
drug addict
drug names
dull pain
duration of pain
dyspnea
elicit
emesis x 5 (emesis times 5)
emotional state
episode
evasive
exacerbated
exacerbations
examinee
excruciating pain
expresses
exquisite pain
extend
fabrication
faint pain
fallacious memories
family background
Family History (FH) section
fan out
feeling (sensation)
feels better when lying down
finesse
flexibility
fluctuating pain
folk medicine
frank
fullness
funny feeling
funny sensation
Gastrointestinal (GI) section
Genitourinary (GU) section
grating sound
grinding sound
grossly inaccurate history
guardian
Habits section
hard of hearing

For Quick Reference

Location of Pain

Physician: Mr. Heaton, can you show me where your pain is right now?

Patient: It's right here. (He points to the left side of his chest, just above the nipple.)

Physician: Does it cover a pretty wide area or is it always right at that spot?

Patient: Always right here.

Physician: Doesn't ever bother you anywhere else in your chest?

Patient: No.

---

sharply circumscribed, confined, delimited, limited, localized

diffuse, ill-defined, nonlocalized, vague

deep in the joint

unilateral headache

Radiation

Physician: . . . or seem to move or spread out from there, into your neck, shoulder, or arm, on either side?

Patient: Hasn't so far.

Physician: Never seems to bore through to your back?

Patient: No.

---

diffuse, extend, fan out, migrate, radiate, spread, wander

bore through, burrow, penetrate, shoot

Duration

Physician: And when did this pain start?

Patient: I noticed it a little bit Sunday night before I went to bed.

Onset

Physician: Did it come on pretty slowly or all of a sudden?

Patient: Just built up slowly Sunday night.

Physician: What were you doing when you first noticed it?

Patient: Reading the paper, I guess. I watched TV a little, too.

Physician: Anyway, you were sitting down, not exerting yourself?

Patient: No.

---

attack, bout, episode, paroxysm, spell of illness

began to develop, came on, developed, started

began to experience, feel, have, note, notice

abrupt, rapid, sudden **onset**   spontaneous

gradual, insidious, slow, subtle **onset**

was healthy, in good health, well until   previously healthy

building up slowly over a period of hours

Intermittency

Physician: Now, has the pain been there ever since it started or does it come and go?

Patient: It stays pretty steady. Of course, I don't notice it when I'm asleep.

constant, persistent, persisting, steady, unabated, unrelenting, unremitting, without letup

coming and going, intermittent, off and on

recurring at odd, random times, long intervals

letting up occasionally

remissions and exacerbations

coming in waves, fluctuating, undulating, waxing and waning

Intensity

Physician: It hasn't kept you awake?

Patient: No.

Physician: Has it been real severe at any time?

Patient: I wouldn't say real severe. I notice it pretty much all the time during the day, but I worked yesterday and today without any trouble.

intensity, severity	mild to moderate pain	faint, mild, slight
interfering with sleep	doubled up with pain	intense, severe

agonizing, crushing, excruciating, exquisite, intolerable, unbearable, unendurable

Quality

Physician: How would you describe the pain? Is it sharp, like a knife stuck in your chest, or dull?

Patient: It's not sharp. Just like a pressure, maybe.

Physician: Not burning?

Patient: No, not really.

ache, aching, discomfort, distress, irritation, misery, pain, rawness, *smarting*, soreness, tickle

pins and needles, prickling, tickling

feeling (sensation): funny, odd, peculiar, strange, uncomfortable, weird

pain: cutting, knifelike, *lancinating*, lightning-like, piercing, ripping, sharp, shooting, sticking, tearing

burning, searing, stinging

feeling: cold, dead, heavy, numb

dull, nagging   feeling, sensation, sense of heat, warmth

pain: boring, pounding, pulsating, splitting, throbbing

sound (sensation): crackling, creaking, grating, grinding, rubbing

compression, constriction, pinching, pressure, squeezing, fullness, heaviness, stiffness, tightness

For Quick Reference

nonlocalized
notions
notoriously
numb feeling
numerous unrelated complaints
obtainable
obtains immediate relief
odd feeling
offense
old records
onset of pain
open
pain aggravated by bending forward
pain at long intervals
pain at random times
pain building up slowly over a period of hours
pain coming and going
pain coming in waves
pain feels worse when up and around
pain interfering with sleep
pain intermittent
pain lets up
pain letting up occasionally
pain lightens up
pain off and on
pain precipitated by deep breathing and coughing
pain recurring at odd times
pain without letup
parent
paroxysm
Past Medical History (PMH) section
pathology
patience
patient
peculiar feeling
penetrate
perceived by the patient
perceptions
persistent pain
persisting pain
personality
physiology
piercing pain
pinching
pins and needles
poor historian
poor intelligence
pounding pain
precipitated
presenting symptom
pressure
previously healthy
prickling
prior episodes
prior illnesses
prior operations

For Quick Reference

Aggravating Factors

Physician: Does it get worse when you take a deep breath, or cough, or move that left arm, or get in certain positions?

Patient: No, it stays pretty much the same.

Physician: Does eating have any effect on it?

Patient: Not that I've noticed. Been eating fine.

> aggravated, brought on, exacerbated, induced, precipitated, provoked, set off, triggered
>
> often precipitated by deep breathing and coughing
>
> aggravated by bending forward, straining at stool
>
> any attempt to move the arm increases pain
>
> feels worse when up and around

Alleviating Factors

Physician: Is there anything that makes it better—lying down, or holding your breath . . . ?

Patient: Seems like if I can burp it feels better for a few minutes.

Physician: Did you take anything for it?

Patient: No. My wife wanted me to take some of her ulcer medicine but I thought I better have you check it out first.

> alleviated, lessened, relieved, mitigated
>
> pain lets up, lightens up
>
> feels better when lying down
>
> breathholding abolishes, relieves pain
>
> obtains immediate, prompt relief
>
> antacids and milk provide temporary relief

Associated Symptoms

Physician: Have you had anything else along with this pain—any shortness of breath, coughing, sweating?

Patient: No.

Physician: And you say your appetite is okay?

Patient: My appetite's fine. Too good.

Physician: Bowels moving okay?

Patient: Okay for me.

Physician: Do you take any medicine regularly? Laxatives, vitamins, any prescription medicine?

Patient: No.

Physician: You mentioned burping. Have you had a lot of burping or gas lately?

Patient: Yes, just since Sunday.

Prior Episodes

Physician: Did you ever have anything like this before?

Patient: I had a pain like this about seven or eight years ago when we used to go to Dr. Abmayer. He said it was indigestion.

Physician: This seems exactly the same?

Patient: Pretty much.

Inciting Factors

Physician: Did you eat anything unusual on Saturday or Sunday?

Patient: We went to a steak house Saturday night and I had one of those things with all the mushrooms and onions on top.

Physician: Has that particular kind of food bothered you before?

Patient: Onions always do.

From the start, the physician had a mental agenda or outline of information to be obtained, but the sequence and wording of the questions depended partly on the way the patient answered. Had the patient been a professor of law or a teenaged girl, the phrasing and even the purport of some of the questions would have been different, even though the same basic range of information was being sought.

The physician's dictation of the part of this patient's history relating to his chief complaint might run something like this:

This 54-year-old white married male toolmaker was well until approximately 48 hours ago when he experienced gradual onset of pain just above the left nipple. The pain is dull, sharply localized, steady, and nonradiating, never severe, not affected by breathing, position, or movement. Belching relieves it temporarily. Pain began about 24 hours after ingestion of a meal with onions at a restaurant. Onions have caused digestive upset in the past, and a similar episode of pain was diagnosed as indigestion by Dr. Abmayer about seven years ago. He has noted belching and flatulence since the pain began but denies dyspnea, diaphoresis, cough, anorexia, nausea, vomiting, or diarrhea and is taking no medicines.

Naturally, chest pain raises different implications and suggests a different line of questioning than, for example, pain in the ear or in the wrist. For each symptom the examiner tries to develop a standard profile of data, giving as full as possible a picture of that symptom in all its dimensions and relations, and providing a basis for comparison with patterns typical of various illnesses.

For Quick Reference

substandard intelligence
sudden onset
symptom
taciturn
tactful interviewer
tangential
tearing pain
tense
throbbing pain
tickle
tickling
tightness
time and effort
triggered
unabated pain
unbearable pain
uncomfortable feeling
uncommunicative
unconsciously
undulating pain
unendurable pain
unilateral headache
unrelenting pain
unreliable
unremitting pain
upset
utmost
vague
ventilates
verbalizes
voices
vomiting
waxing and waning pain
weird feeling (sensation)
well-being
withdrawn
written records

Exercises for Chapter 1

Review and Summarize

A. Multiple Choice

___ 1. According to the text, a patient whose history appears vague or unreliable may be labeled
  a. Demented.
  b. Uncooperative.
  c. Belligerent.
  d. A poor historian.

___ 2. Factors such as the informant's memory and ability to communicate, intelligence, and willingness to cooperate affect the history-taking by
  a. Limiting the volume and validity of the history.
  b. Creating an unnecessarily lengthy history.
  c. Deliberately confusing the history taker.
  d. Causing all information contained in the history to be questionable.

B. Fill in the Blank

1. When the patient is unable to provide an accurate history or any history at all, the physician may obtain the

  patient's history from _____.

2. The _____ of the medical history depends on the reason for

  obtaining it, the patient's condition and ability to communicate, and other factors.

C. Short Answer

1. According to the text, what factors affect the information obtained during history-taking?

  _____

  _____

  _____

  _____

  _____

2. Write a short definition of the following terms. If you can, condense the definition into just a few words or a single synonym that you feel more comfortable with. Note that some words are not medical words. Their application to the medical context may be different from their use in other contexts and may take some extrapolation on your part.

a. Adamantly _____

b. Alleges _____

c. Tangential _____

d. Logorrhea _____

e. Confabulates_____

f. Perseverates _____

g. Mendacious_____

h. Delimited _____

i. Insidious _____

j. Unabated _____

k. Unremitting _____

l. Fluctuating _____

m. Exquisite _____

n. Mitigated _____

o. Inciting _____

Pause and Reflect

Have you ever accompanied an elderly person to a physician's office or hospital? Were you present during the interview and examination? (If not, try to imagine such a situation with an elderly person you may know.) Describe the interview. What factors discussed at the beginning of this chapter affected the history-taking by the medical personnel and the history-giving by the patient? How accurate and extensive a history was obtained? Which of the vocabulary terms noted in the chapter related to the interview?

_____

_____

_____

_____

_____

_____

_____

_____

Explain and Learn

Turn to the person next to you (or behind or in front of you), and share with each other one important piece of information you got from this chapter. Also share how you might use this information in your life or in your work. If you have a question that wasn't answered in the chapter, share that as well. If your partner doesn't have the answer, ask your instructor.

Relax and Play

Using the words from the list in the Short Answer questions or at least 10 terms from the word list in the chapter, write a poem or song that incorporates these terms in such a way as to reveal their meaning or use. If writing a song, use a familiar tune or rap style.

Generalize and Apply

In your book, using the "dictated summary" of the physician's interview with the patient and the headings for the description of the interview ("Location of Pain," "Radiation," and so on), draw lines from relevant words or phrases in the dictated summary and label with the appropriate heading.

Collaborate and Share

Consider the following statement made at the end of the chapter: "For each symptom the examiner tries to develop a standard profile of data, giving as full as possible a picture of that symptom in all its dimensions and relations, and providing a basis for comparison with patterns typical of various illnesses." Discuss how this statement is reflected in the interview of the patient with chest pain. Give specific examples.

_____

_____

_____

_____

Relate and Remember

A metaphor is like a picture story: One thing, not necessarily similar, represents something else. For example, an ice cube might be a visual metaphor for waiting in a doctor's office. As it melts, both patience and energy disappear into a puddle of annoyance and despair. "It's raining cats and dogs" is an example of a verbal metaphor. Metaphors can help us learn in two ways: One, by helping us remember a fact or point we associate with the metaphor; two, by helping us to look at a point from a different angle or point of view.

Think of a metaphor that completes this statement: Obtaining an accurate and complete patient history is like a _____. Use a visual or a verbal metaphor. Fill in the blank with the name of an object or draw (or cut out of a magazine) a picture representing one or more important points. Explain your choice in light of the discussion at the beginning of the chapter.

_____

_____

_____

_____

_____

_____

_____

_____

_____

Extrapolate and Project

A mind map is a visual method of note-taking. It's much more fun than outlining and can be more effective in helping you to remember the important details of something you've read or heard in a lecture. Mind maps use graphic or pictorial ways to show the relationships between one fact and another or one idea and another. These relationships may be displayed, for example, like a family tree, a pie graph, a chart, a spreadsheet, or in any number of other ways. This technique will be referred to in future exercises.

The drawing below is a mind map which is partially completed. Inside the 12 exterior circles, write the chest pain parameters about which the doctor asked the patient (the headings used in the interview description—radiation, location, duration, etc.). From each of these, draw two additional lines with circles. Label one circle + (positives) and one - (negatives) and enter the terms that apply. For example, for the positive circle linked to location, you would enter "above nipple," in the negative circle "nowhere else." After you have displayed all the patient's positive and negative symptoms this way, look at your drawing. Does it help you to see relationships better? Are there more positive or negative responses? Do you think the patient has cardiac (heart) or noncardiac (musculoskeletal, pulmonary, or gastrointestinal) chest pain? Why? Now that the physician has clearly defined the patient's pain, what do you think the next step would be?

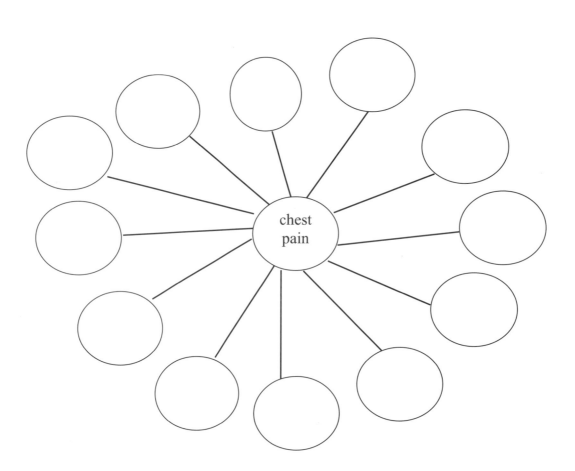

2

Chief Complaint and History of Present Illness

The statement of the patient's chief (or presenting) complaint (or complaints) and a narration of the course of the illness up to the moment when the history is taken far outweigh the rest of the history in importance. In fact, the other parts of the history may be dealt with perfunctorily or even omitted altogether in the case of a simple, clear-cut illness or injury. There is almost no limit to the variety of problems that can induce a person to seek medical attention. A detailed cataloging of possible chief complaints is beyond the scope of this chapter. Discussions of many common complaints are presented in Chapters 7 through 14, which cover the Review of Systems. The pediatric history and physical examination are discussed in Chapter 29.

CC (Chief Complaint)

presenting complaint

principal complaint

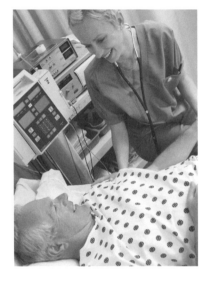

Some physicians prefer to state the Chief Complaint exactly in the patient's words ("I can't sleep," "My left arm is numb"), while others strive for maximum conciseness and precision ("Insomnia," "Hypesthesia of the dorsum of the left forearm"). Often the statement of the chief complaint includes an indication of its duration or other features: "Intermittent pain and pressure in the epigastrium for one week." Sometimes several apparently related complaints are mentioned together: "Fever, vomiting, diarrhea, and severe headache." Even when the patient cannot give any history, the heading "Chief Complaint" is still used: "Sudden loss of consciousness at home and deepening coma."

The History of Present Illness (HPI) is the heart of the medical history, for it contains all historical details leading up to and in any way pertaining to the patient's current status. If, for example, a patient is hospitalized for pneumonia, the History of Present Illness might include mention of smoking habits, current medicines, previous treatments or hospitalizations for respiratory disease, and all negative and positive answers to questions about the respiratory tract, even though this material would probably appear in other parts of the history if the patient had appendicitis instead of pneumonia. In an acute illness, the History of Present Illness may consist of just a sentence or two, but if the patient's current problem is the culmination of months or years of chronic, evolving illness, this part of the history may occupy a whole page or more.

The narrative of the course of an illness follows a certain pattern, basically chronologic. By convention, the physician starts with a brief description of the

Learning Objectives

After careful study of this chapter, you should be able to:

Define the phrase *chief complaint* and give examples of the different ways a Chief Complaint can be expressed.

Discuss the scope of the History of Present Illness.

Explain why it is difficult to pinpoint the exact origin of an illness.

Propose questions to elicit the severity of symptoms.

List general symptoms that occur in a variety of conditions.

Give examples of actions patients may take in an attempt to restore their own health.

Describe the organization of information within the History of Present Illness.

For Quick Reference

patient, including age and sex and often race and social status, then records the date (or time) and nature of onset of the first symptoms and traces the progress of the illness—the appearance of additional symptoms, their effect on the patient's lifestyle and well-being, and the results of treatment, physician-prescribed or otherwise—finally reporting the events that prompted the present consultation or hospitalization. This part of the history may contain an almost limitless variety of information, including diagnoses and the names of drugs and operations, which cannot be considered here.

> This 31-year-old housewife *presented* to the emergency room on New Year's Day with the complaint of severe flank pain, chills, and fever.
>
> This is the third Collins Annex admission of this 44-year-old white retarded male for status epilepticus.
>
> This 86-year-old African-American woman is admitted from Garden Nursing Home because of dehydration and change in mental status.
>
> This 45-year-old married mother of 3 children first noted a 2.5 x 2.5 cm hard, irregular, nontender mass in the upper outer quadrant of the left breast about 6 weeks ago.
>
> This 81-year-old male has had a 3-year history of feeling that he has lost balance, woozy spells, light-headedness, and some suggestion of true vertigo, but he is less certain of this latter symptomatology.

In narrating the History of Present Illness, the physician usually gives some indication of the patient's general state of health before the onset of symptoms. The present illness may arise from some preexisting or predisposing condition or may represent a complication or exacerbation of a chronic problem. Previous hospitalizations or operations or long-term medications may deserve mention.

> This 20-year-old single white male student was essentially well until Friday morning, when he awakened with fever and headache.
>
> The patient had several prior episodes of nausea, vomiting, and right upper quadrant pain.
>
> The patient is a known diabetic *maintained* for about 4 years on diet and an oral agent.
>
> Seizures have been well controlled on Depakote.
>
> previously healthy adult female   was asymptomatic, essentially well until

A general decline in energy level or sense of well-being may be the only clue to the onset of illness. The patient may say "I haven't felt up to par" or "I'm not my usual self lately." Nonspecific symptoms such as fever, chills, loss of appetite,

> has felt generally unwell for about 4 weeks
>
> reduced exercise tolerance
>
> draggy, exhausted, run down, sluggish, tired, washed out, wiped out, worn out
>
> asthenia, easy fatigability, fatigue, languor, lassitude, listlessness, malaise, prostration, tiredness, weakness
>
> generalized aching, myalgia   vague aches and pains

headaches, muscle aches, lethargy, drowsiness, decline in exercise tolerance, and inability to concentrate can herald the onset of a broad variety of diseases.

The beginning of an illness is often extremely subtle, so that days or weeks may go by before even the patient becomes aware that this is more than a passing indisposition. Two or more symptoms occurring at the same time may seem at first to be unrelated, their connection or common origin becoming apparent only when they evolve, worsen, or become complicated by further trouble. Again, unrelated symptoms occurring together may seem to be part of a single problem. Hence, it is sometimes nearly impossible to pin down the date of origin of an illness or to reconstruct the chronology from what the patient remembers.

No matter what the initial or presenting symptom, the physician will try to learn when it started; whether it came on gradually or abruptly; whether it has continued unchanged, waxed and waned, or intermittently disappeared; and whether the patient can suggest any reason for it. The duration of a symptom is of the utmost importance in analyzing its meaning. A 12-hour history of constant, agonizing, unilateral headache with blurred vision and vomiting might indicate cerebral hemorrhage, encephalitis, meningitis, or brain abscess, among other possibilities. A 20-year history of such headaches recurring at intervals could not possibly be due to any of these. Similarly, the suddenness with which a symptom appears and the pattern of its subsequent behavior may supply essential clues to its significance.

> began to develop, came on, developed, started   spontaneous
>
> began to experience, feel, have, note, notice
>
> **onset**: abrupt, acute, gradual, insidious, rapid, slow, sudden, subtle
>
> chronic, constant, longstanding, persistent, persisting, steady, unabated, unrelenting, unremitting, without letup

Patients frequently relate the beginning of an illness to some action or event that occurred a short time before the first symptoms appeared. Explanations offered by patients for the origins of their symptoms are too often correct for any of them to be safely ignored by the physician. On the other hand, such explanations may be based on utterly naïve concepts of pathophysiology or may arise from feelings of guilt or resentment. For instance, a patient who has had an extramarital affair may interpret a case of ringworm as evidence of sexually transmitted infection. The victim of an accidental injury at work may half-sincerely blame all subsequent medical problems on that one distressing incident.

Assessing the severity of symptoms sometimes poses great difficulties. A stoic patient plays down medical troubles; a hypochondriac exaggerates them. Determining what effect symptoms have had on daily life and normal activities may provide a useful yardstick. Has the illness caused occupational disability? Have social

> has been able to carry on, continue with normal daily activities
>
> has missed, been absent from work, school
>
> has been staying home
>
> unable to do her usual housework
>
> ADLs (activities of daily living)

For Quick Reference

exhausted
extramarital affair
failed chemotherapy
family relationships
fatigue
feeling flushed
feelings of guilt or resentment
felt generally unwell
fever
flu-like symptoms
fluid retention
flushing
followed
gender
generalized aching
gradual onset
grippe
grippy feeling
hard mass
headaches recurring at intervals
healthy adult female
high fever
historical details
History of the Present Illness (HPI)
home remedies
hospitalization
hot flashes
hot flushes
hot spells
hyperhidrosis
hypertension
hypochondriac
increased appetite
increasing dyspnea
increasing pain
initial symptom
insidious onset
irregular mass
known diabetic
languor
lassitude
leftover antibiotic capsules
lifestyle
light-headedness
listlessness
longstanding
loss of appetite
lost balance
low grade fever
maintenance dose
malaise
malignancy
mass in upper outer quadrant of breast
meaning of symptoms
medical attention
medical history
meningitis
mental illness

For Quick Reference

or recreational activities had to be canceled or modified? Have family relationships and obligations suffered?

Certain general symptoms occur in such a variety of conditions that they often receive mention, if only negatively, in the History of Present Illness. Fever, manifested by an uncomfortable sensation of excessive warmth, flushing, or sweating, especially at night, usually indicates infection but can arise from systemic disease or malignancy. Chills, varying from a sensation of coolness to violent shivering, seldom occur without fever and likewise usually indicate infection. The appetite serves as a reliable barometer of health, seldom remaining unaffected in serious illness. Appetite, digestion, and bowel function may all suffer disturbance together. Subtle loss of appetite that escapes even the patient's notice will eventually be betrayed by loss of weight. Gain of weight not explainable by change of diet usually signifies fluid retention. Sleeping habits are likewise sensitive indicators of illness, both physical and mental.

> **fever**: high, low grade, mild, slight, spiking
>
> feeling flushed, hot, sweaty, warm
>
> fever, flushing, hot flashes, hot flushes, hot spells, warmth
>
> diaphoresis, hyperhidrosis
>
> copious, drenching sweats   night sweats
>
> chills, rigors, shaking chills, shivering
>
> flu-like symptoms, grippe, grippy feeling
>
> Appetite, digestion, and bowel habits have remained unaffected and weight is stable.
>
> anorexia, diminished appetite, reduced appetite, loss of appetite
>
> bulimia, increased appetite, polyphagia
>
> ravenous, voracious hunger
>
> polydipsia, (excessive) thirst
>
> He has lost some weight and notes that his clothes feel loose.
>
> He has lost about 10 pounds in the past few weeks.

The typical patient doesn't wait long after the appearance of symptoms before taking some action against them. This may include changing the usual pattern of living or diet to avoid aggravating the problem, applying various home remedies, using prescription medicines left over from a previous illness, or consulting a physician. The effect, if any, of various attempts to restore normal health and functioning may provide valuable sidelights on the character, severity, or meaning of symptoms. Previous diagnoses, prescribed medicines, and operations can all contribute to an understanding of the present illness. Patients are often extremely vague

> drug, medication, medicine, remedy
>
> OTC (over-the-counter), patent, *proprietary medicine*
>
> He took a proprietary cough preparation for several days without relief.
>
> She borrowed some yellow tablets from her girlfriend, who takes them for asthma.
>
> She has been taking some leftover antibiotic capsules erratically for 3 or 4 days.
>
> He has been on a green nerve pill for several weeks.

He was *worked up* by me approximately 8 months ago for hypertension.

He has been *followed* by Dr. Wilson.

on *steroids*   *chronic* anticonvulsant therapy

He was placed, put, started on chlorothiazide 2 years ago but *compliance* has evidently been poor.

He achieved good control on a maintenance dose of 25 mg t.i.d.

dose was adjusted, *titrated, tapered, weaned*

refractory to medical management

failed chemotherapy

She underwent triple coronary bypass on March 18.

as to what medicines they have been taking and how they have been taking them. They may also incorrectly report diagnoses made by other physicians, or be unable to state clearly how these diagnoses were established.

The physician usually carries the History of Present Illness down to the present by describing the circumstances in which the patient sought medical attention. At this point, all historical data considered relevant to the patient's present condition have been recorded. By convention, however, the examiner proceeds to review, in orderly fashion, other aspects of the patient's medical history, both for the sake of completeness and because unsuspected clues and relationships are frequently uncovered in the process. These further divisions of the history are discussed in Chapters 3 through 14.

Because of increasing pain and dyspnea he was brought by his wife to St. Luke's Medical Center Emergency Department about 4 o'clock this morning.

For Quick Reference

slow onset
sluggish
smoking habits
social activities
social status of patient
spiking fever
spontaneous
stable weight
status epilepticus
steady
stoic patient
subsequent behavior
subsequent medical problems
subtle loss of appetite
subtle onset
sudden onset
sudden symptom
suddenness
sweating
sweaty
symptomatology
systemic disease
tapered
tiredness
triple coronary bypass
true vertigo
typical patient
unabated
unable to do her usual housework
unaffected
underwent triple coronary bypass
unilateral headache
unrelenting
unremitting
unsuspected clues
unsuspected relationships
upper outer quadrant of breast
upper quadrant pain
vague aches and pains
violent shivering
vomiting
voracious hunger
washed out
weakness
weaned
weight stable
well-being
wiped out
without letup
woozy spells
worn out
yardstick

Exercises for Chapter 2

Review and Summarize

A. Multiple Choice

___ 1. Some parts of the medical history may be omitted but never the
    a. Review of Systems.
    b. Family History.
    c. History of Present Illness.
    d. Past Surgical History.

___ 2. The patient's own words may be used to describe the
    a. Chief Complaint.
    b. History of Present Illness.
    c. Family History.
    d. Social History.

B. Fill in the Blank

1. The _____ and _____, which may be combined,

   far outweigh the rest of the history in importance.

2. The _____ is the heart of the medical history.

3. The narrative pattern of the History of Present Illness is, usually, _____.

4. The _____ of a symptom is of utmost importance in analyzing its meaning.

C. Short Answer

1. Why is the History of Present Illness so important?

   _____

   _____

   _____

2. What factors make it difficult if not impossible to pin down the date of origin or reconstruct the chronology of a patient's illness?

   _____

   _____

3. Write a short definition of the following terms. If you can, condense the definition into just a few words or a single synonym that you feel more comfortable with. Note that some words are not medical words. Their application to the medical context may be different from their use in other contexts and may take some extrapolation on your part.

a. Perfunctorily _____

b. Principal _____

c. Preexisting condition _____

d. Predisposing condition _____

e. Exacerbation _____

f. Indisposition _____

g. Asthenia _____

h. Languor _____

i. Malaise _____

j. Proprietary _____

k. Compliance _____

l. Refractory _____

Pause and Reflect

Think about a significant illness you or someone close to you has had. Describe what might have appeared in the Chief Complaint and History of Present Illness.

_____

_____

_____

_____

_____

_____

_____

_____

_____

Relate and Remember

Read the paragraph beginning "The narrative of the course of an illness follows a certain pattern..." Three steps are mentioned, beginning with the words "starts," "then," and "finally." Draw a mind map using "course of illness" as the main point and these three points as the key points from which you will build the remainder of the map. A design like a family tree for this exercise would work well, but you can use any visual pattern that works for you. From each of the three main "branches," list specific factors included in that branch. In the following paragraphs, the patient's condition prior to the onset of the illness, the timing of the onset of the symptoms, the duration of the symptoms, the severity of the symptoms, the presence or absence of generalized nonspecific symptoms, and the circumstances which caused the patient to seek treatment are discussed. Add these topics and relevant details relating to them to your map. Can you now visualize the structure and extent of a narrative History of Present Illness? Could you take this map and fill in details relating to a specific illness? Try this with an illness with which you are familiar.

Collaborate and Share

With a partner, role-play doctor and patient, taking each role in turn. As doctor, interview the patient using the information you've gained in the introduction and first two chapters of this book. Take notes. As patient, use the presenting complaint and course of an illness you or someone close to you has actually had. After each of you has played both doctor and patient, type on a separate sheet or handwrite below the Chief Complaint and History of Present Illness for the patient you interviewed.

_____

_____

_____

_____

_____

Explain and Learn

List some of the symptoms that are an indication of illness but are so generalized, appearing with a variety of illnesses, that their presence does not necessarily help elucidate the cause of the illness. Why are they important? Present your answer to the class, to a partner, or a group as directed by your instructor.

_____

_____

_____

_____

_____

_____

_____

_____

_____

Generalize and Apply

What determines whether information appears in the History of Present Illness or somewhere else in the medical history report? Give examples.

_____

_____

_____

_____

_____

_____

_____

_____

_____

_____

_____

_____

Extrapolate and Project

Explain the importance of an accurate History of Present Illness. What might be the consequence of omitted, fabricated, or erroneous details? Give examples. You may use examples from your own experience.

_____

_____

_____

_____

_____

_____

_____

_____

_____

_____

_____

_____

_____

_____

3

Family History

The importance of the Family History lies in the fact that many developmental abnormalities, diseases, and tendencies to disease are not only hereditary (genetically transmitted from parent to child) but familial (occurring in some or all members of a family). In addition, a thorough family history can provide clues to unwholesome environmental influences or exposure to communicable disease.

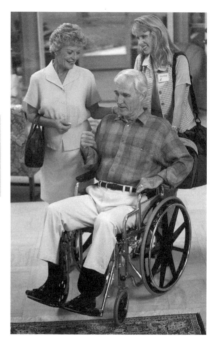

Family History: Noncontributory, Unremarkable

Patient was adopted and has no information about the health of his biologic (natural, real) parents.

The complete Family History includes the age and state of health (or age at death and cause of death) of each member of the patient's immediate family (parents, siblings, and children), selected data about other blood relatives, and a general statement regarding family history of certain conditions. In practice the Family History is often passed over as noncontributory or irrelevant, and sometimes it is omitted altogether. Part or all of it may be assumed into the Social History.

Both parents and two sisters are living and well. A brother died in infancy of unknown cause.

Maternal grandmother and one of three maternal aunts had type 2 diabetes mellitus.

His father died at age 54 of MI. His mother is 71 and in fair health except for arthritis of the spine and hips. One brother, aged 49, has angina, and another, aged 44, has high blood pressure.

Patient's parents were divorced when he was 11. His mother was hospitalized several times for mental illness both before and after the divorce.

There is no family history of heart disease, hypertension, diabetes, sickle cell anemia, tuberculosis, cancer, asthma, or arthritis.

The patient reports a strong family history of alcoholism and drug-related problems.

Family history is negative for hypertension, abnormal serum lipids, and diabetes.

Mother has insulin-dependent diabetes, but the siblings do not have any problems with polyuria, even though they get up about once a night to void. There is also a history of recurrent UTIs in the mother and the maternal grandfather.

Learning Objectives

After careful study of this chapter, you should be able to:

Explain the importance of the Family History to the diagnostic process.

Distinguish between *hereditary* and *familial* conditions.

List the components of a complete Family History.

Given statements from a patient history, identify those that are related to the Family History.

Exercises for Chapter 3

Review and Summarize

A. Multiple Choice

___ 1. A disease that occurs in some or all members of a family is called
    a. Familiar.
    b. Familial.
    c. Familism.
    d. Familiarized.

___ 2. The patient's immediate family includes
    a. Spouse, parents, children.
    b. Brothers, sisters, cousins.
    c. Aunts, uncles, siblings.
    d. Parents, siblings, children.

___ 3. Part of the Family History may be included in the
    a. Social History.
    b. Review of Systems.
    c. Chief Complaint.
    d. Past Medical History.

B. Short Answer

1. List the reasons why the Family History is an important part of the patient's medical record.

    _____

    _____

2. Identify the type of information included in the Family History.

    _____

    _____

3. Define *sibling*.

    _____

4. Define *hereditary*.

    _____

Pause and Reflect

Type on a separate sheet or handwrite below your family history as though it were a part of your medical record. Are there any inherited diseases in your family? Do members of your family have a tendency to certain illnesses (like hypertension, obesity, mental illness)? Are there any factors in your family history that relate to illnesses you have had? Note: This exercise is for practice only and should not be turned in as it may contain personal information you may not wish to share.

_____

_____

_____

_____

Collaborate and Share

Combine your knowledge of various diseases. List as many hereditary (genetic) and familial diseases as you can based on your personal experience or studies. Share your list with the rest of the class.

_____

_____

_____

_____

_____

Explain and Learn

If you are very familiar with a hereditary disease, share what you know about this disease with the other members of the class, or handwrite below. What causes it? What are the symptoms and signs of the disease? What is the treatment? Can it be cured?

_____

_____

_____

_____

_____

Extrapolate and Project

1. If an adoptee has no access to the medical histories of birth parents, speculate on other ways to get this information.

_____

_____

_____

_____

2. Find an article that describes and explains the Human Genome Project. Without getting into controversy over the ethical or nonethical uses of this information, what changes do you foresee in the diagnosis and treatment of hereditary as well as nonhereditary diseases?

_____

_____

_____

_____

4

Social History

This part of the history includes any personal information about the patient's past or present life that, although nonmedical, may have a bearing on health. The ideal Social History would include data on the patient's birth, upbringing, academic career, marital history and present status, spouse's health history, military service, occupations past and present, avocations and hobbies, social and cultural pursuits, political and religious activities, foreign travel or residence, financial status, police record, and current family structure, living arrangements, and personal responsibilities.

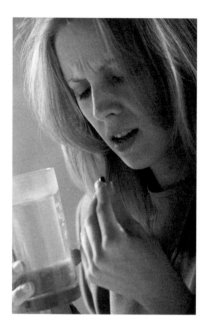

> Married. Retired. Five children. Does not smoke; quit about 12 years ago. Drinks alcohol, one cup of wine at dinner.
>
> The patient is retired. Smoking and alcohol abuse denied.
>
> The patient is a 17-year-old I.V. drug abuser.
>
> Widowed, two children. Smokes one pack of cigarettes per day.

Seldom does the physician have time or motivation to extract such a voluminous mass of nonmedical and doubtfully relevant information from a patient, except in the course of psychotherapy. Hence the Social History is often omitted, a brief note of the patient's age, marital status, and occupation having been inserted in the History of Present Illness. Other elements of the Social History may also appear in the History of Present Illness. For example, the occupational history of a patient with hearing loss, dermatitis, or asthma may be highly relevant to the diagnosis. A history of travel in the tropics can lead to the explanation of an unusual case of fever or diarrhea.

A complete occupational history includes dates of all jobs held by the patient, with attention to exposure to hazardous chemicals, noise, psychological stress, and other adverse conditions; industrial illnesses or injuries, workers' compensation claims filed, and disability allowances; medical or other restrictions on work assignments; use of safety devices such as hearing protection and goggles; moonlighting or overtime; and satisfaction with current job. A job title or classification may need to be supplemented by a detailed explanation of duties, environmental stresses, and hazards.

Learning Objectives

After careful study of this chapter, you should be able to:

Explain the role of the Social History in the diagnostic process.

Characterize an ideal Social History.

Given statements from a patient history, identify those that are related to Social History.

List the components of a complete occupational history.

Justify a physician's omission of the Social History.

Exercises for Chapter 4

Review and Summarize

A. Multiple Choice

___ 1. Which of the following would NOT be classified under Social History?
   a. Psychiatric history.
   b. Travel history.
   c. Occupational history.
   d. Financial status.

___ 2. Elements of the Social History may also appear in the
   a. Mental status exam.
   b. History of Present Illness.
   c. Spouse's health history.
   d. Review of Systems.

B. Short Answer

List the elements that might be included in a complete Social History.

_____

_____

_____

Pause and Reflect

Using the list above, type on a separate sheet or handwrite below your own Social History as it might appear in a medical record.

_____

_____

_____

_____

_____

Generalize and Apply

Using the list above, draw a mind map. For each of the different elements of the Social History, list as many disease conditions as you can that might be relevant to that element. For example, under employment history, having worked in a factory that processes asbestos would be relevant to asbestosis.

Extrapolate and Project

Complete social histories are rarely included except in a psychiatric report, and abbreviated information may be included in the History of Present Illness instead. Indeed, psychiatric nurses and social workers are often the ones to compile and dictate the social history on a mentally ill patient, and it may be several pages long. Why do you think a complete Social History would be more relevant to a psychiatric report? What elements listed above might, in your opinion, be most important? Why?

_____

_____

_____

_____

_____

_____

_____

5

Habits

Under this heading comes information about the patient's regular or customary practices with respect to eating, sleeping, exercise, recreation, and the use of prescription and nonprescription medicines, caffeine, nicotine, alcohol, and other substances of abuse—in a word, the patient's lifestyle. The physician may choose not to explore some of these sensitive and private matters until close rapport has been established with the patient, unless they seem likely to have a direct bearing on the patient's current health status.

> Habits: Drinks 3 to 4 cups of coffee a day and smokes 1 to $1^1/_2$ packs of cigarettes a day.
> Denies any use of prescription medicines or illicit drugs.

Dietary habits need to be investigated if the patient has a weight problem or digestive tract symptoms. A full dietary history covers the number of meals taken daily; regularity of mealtimes; circumstances of eating; composition and balance of meals as to fats, carbohydrates, and proteins; any self-imposed dietary restrictions (fad or weight-reduction diets, religious abstinence, vegetarianism); snacking, bingeing, and fasting practices; weight history; use of dietary supplements, health foods, and vitamins; and an estimate of average daily caloric intake. Persons with eating disorders (anorexia nervosa, bulimia nervosa) seldom give accurate accounts of their dietary practices.

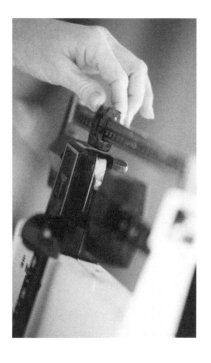

> eats three meals a day   vegetarian, vegan
> erratic, irregular eating habits   fasting, dieting   fast foods, snacks
> The most he has ever weighed is 225 lb.
> follows an 1800-calorie ADA diet

The sleep history includes hours of sleep each night, ease of falling asleep, tendency to awaken during the night, restfulness of sleep, use of sleeping medicines, daytime napping, nightmares, and sleepwalking.

> gets about 6 hours' sleep each night   insomnia, sleeplessness
> has difficulty falling asleep
> awakens before dawn and cannot get back to sleep
> hypnotic, sedative, sleeping pills   nightmares
> sleepwalking, somnambulism

Learning Objectives

After careful study of this chapter, you should be able to:

Define the term *habits* in the context of a patient's medical history.

Describe the components of a full dietary history.

Identify terms related to the sleep history.

Explain lifestyle clues that relate to a patient's exercise, reaction, and vacation habits.

Name the five components of a satisfactory medication record.

Discuss the problems a physician may encounter in eliciting a history of drug or alcohol abuse.

For Quick Reference

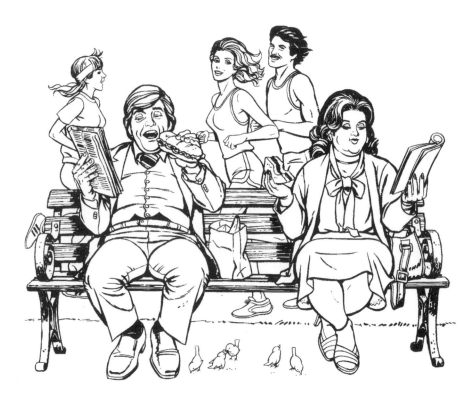

A person's habits regarding exercise, recreations, and vacations from work may supply clues to risk-taking, compulsive, or excessively sedentary lifestyles.

describes himself as a workaholic

Besides coffee and tea, many soft drinks (particularly of the cola variety), herbal teas, and chocolate contain caffeine or caffeine-like stimulants.

Denies coffee, tea, or cola beverages.

A useful unit for recording lifetime cigarette smoking history is the *pack-year*, which is the equivalent of smoking one package of cigarettes a day for one year. Hence a person who smoked $1\frac{1}{2}$ packages of cigarettes a day for 24 years would be called a 36-pack-year smoker.

chain smoker   dips snuff   uses smokeless tobacco   chews tobacco
smokes approximately $2\frac{1}{2}$ packs of cigarettes daily and inhales
He stopped smoking after his first infarct. He had a 50-pack-year history.

It is desirable to compile, as a part of every patient's history, a complete list of all prescription and nonprescription medicines presently being taken, including ointments, eye or nose drops, inhalers, and patches, as well as of medicines taken irregularly for specific indications. Patients are often unable to tell the names or purposes of medicines prescribed for them by physicians. In addition, it is difficult at times to judge how well a forgetful or confused person has been adhering to a therapeutic regimen. Many persons do not think of oral contraceptives, vitamin

drinks in moderation

admits heavy social drinking on weekends

admits frequent solitary drinking

drinks 2 or 3 beers each evening

has consumed approximately 1 pint of whiskey daily for 6 years

has a 10-year history of alcoholism, ethanolism, alcohol dependency

supplements, laxatives, and headache and cold remedies as medicines, and must be closely questioned before recalling and reporting their use. A satisfactory record of medicine use should include the name—preferably the generic name—of each medicine, the dosage form, strength, and frequency of use, and the purpose for which it was prescribed.

Persons who abuse alcohol or drugs are notoriously unreliable historians. The more searching the interrogation, the more likely they are to conceal or distort the truth about their drinking or drug use and other elements of their health history that may be in any way related to it. Queries about the type and volume of alcoholic beverages consumed yield much the same answers whether the patient drinks a little or a lot. When alcohol abuse is suspected, questions that may supply important evidence are those concerning drinking alone, drinking in the morning to get started or to stop shaking, blackouts or spells of amnesia, arrests for public drunkenness or drunk driving, and the effects of drinking on work, family, and social relationships. A problem drinker may give false or misleading answers to all such questions, particularly when the physician has no other source of information.

Although drug abusers characteristically conceal the details of their drug-taking, the fear of death may render them voluble. Unfortunately, abusers of street drugs often know them by names that convey no information about their composition to the physician. Besides drugs as such, a number of household and industrial chemicals—adhesives, solvents, and aerosol propellants—are subject to recreational abuse. Intravenous drug abuse, with sharing of a needle by several persons, frequently results in transmission of infectious diseases, particularly hepatitis B and AIDS.

occasional recreational drug use

smokes marijuana approximately 4 times a week

I.V. (intravenous) drug abuse

Exercises for Chapter 5

Review and Summarize

A. Multiple Choice

___1. The report of a patient's habits may include all of the following EXCEPT
   a. Dietary habits.
   b. Bowel habits.
   c. Smoking or drinking habits.
   d. Sleeping habits.
   e. Medications.

___2. Of the following types of patients, which are likely to be the *most* unreliable when giving the history of their habits?
   a. Obese patients.
   b. Sedentary patients.
   c. Elderly patients.
   d. Alcohol or drug abusers.
   e. Children.

B. Fill in the Blank

1. The recording of a patient's usual or customary habits is, in short, a reflection of the patient's

   _____.

2. Soft drinks, herbal teas, and chocolate consumption are relevant to the patient's _____

   intake.

3. Persons with _____ seldom give an accurate history of their dietary habits.

4. Persons who abuse _____ or _____ are notoriously

   unreliable historians.

5. A unit for recording lifetime cigarette smoking history is the _____.

6. A complete medication includes a list of all _____

   and _____ medications being taken by the patient.

C. Short Answer

1. List the types of prescription and nonprescription medications a patient might take. What might patients omit from their medication history because they don't see them as medicines? What should be included in a satisfactory record of medicine use?

_____

_____

_____

_____

_____

_____

2. A reliable history is difficult to obtain from patients who abuse alcohol. What are some of the clues to excessive alcohol use?

_____

_____

3. Write a short definition of the following terms. If you can, condense the definition into just a few words or a single synonym that you feel more comfortable with. Note that some of these words are not medical words. Their application to the medical context may be different from their use in other contexts and may take some extrapolation on your part.

a. Abstinence _____

b. Anorexia nervosa _____

c. Bulimia nervosa _____

d. Insomnia_____

e. Somnambulism_____

f. Sedentary _____

g. Voluble _____

h. Ethanolism_____

i. Pack-year_____

Pause and Reflect

Type on a separate sheet or handwrite below your own Habits history as it might appear in a medical record.

_____

_____

_____

_____

_____

_____

Relate and Remember

Draw a mind map or family tree to illustrate the elements that are included under Habits in the medical history. From the primary subtopics (diet, exercise, substance abuse, etc.), add the details pertinent to that topic.

Collaborate and Share

Using the mind map or tree created above, list some of the disease conditions that might be relevant to the different elements; for example, liver disease related to excessive alcohol abuse. Share with the rest of the class.

_____

_____

_____

_____

Generalize and Apply

Discuss the relevance of Habits to illness and disease processes. What habits might be major factors, which ones minor? Give examples.

_____

_____

_____

Extrapolate and Project

In the activities for the last chapter, you discussed the effects of heredity on disease and how genetic research might influence health in the future. In view of the effects of a person's lifestyle and environment on illness and disease, do you see a time when most illnesses might be cured? Why or why not? What medical research is being done in the area of lifestyle influences on disease? What types of changes do you think are needed (globally or individually) to reduce or eliminate diseases related to lifestyle factors? Write down and share your comments with the rest of the class.

_____

_____

_____

_____

_____

_____

6

Past Medical History: General

The Past Medical History (PMH) provides a concluding survey of all medical information not covered in any previous section of the history. The inclusion of material here implies that it is not considered relevant to the History of Present Illness. Hence the Past Medical History may be run through, or at least recorded, in perfunctory fashion, and may consist largely of negatives. ("The remainder of the history is negative.") The format of the present book calls for a more elaborate discussion of historical points in the Past Medical History, and particularly in the Review of Systems (next chapter), than would ever be found in an actual history.

The general medical history is conventionally discussed under the headings of Past Illnesses, Past Injuries, Surgical Operations, Chronic Diseases and Disabilities, Allergies, and Immunizations. For the sake of continuity, these boundaries may be ignored. For example, it makes better sense to discuss an injury, its surgical treatment, any resulting current disability, and medicines presently being taken because of it in a continuous narrative than to fragment the subject according to a set of artificial divisions.

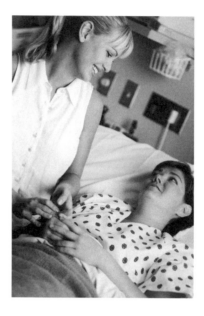

Past Illnesses

This part of the history reports past episodes or attacks of clearly defined, named diseases. When asked to recall all prior illnesses, most of us perform poorly. The physician's customary strategy is to list ten to twenty common, serious diseases (diabetes, tuberculosis, asthma, pneumonia, high blood pressure, heart attack or heart disease, stroke, epilepsy, ulcer, cancer, anemia, arthritis, kidney disease, nervous or mental disease) and ask whether the patient has had any of them. An affirmative answer prompts inquiries about dates, severity, treatment, complications, or sequelae. Sometimes asking about hospitalizations rather than about illnesses yields a better return. Often the patient's recollections must be supplemented or corrected by reference to written records. The frequency with which "old" hospital charts and medical files, when they can be obtained, supply crucial historical data should give all health professionals continuing motivation to keep full and accurate records.

> past, previous, prior, remote history of peptic ulcer
> *documented* cirrhosis
> without complications or *sequelae*   *residuals*
> several *episodes* of pancreatitis

Learning Objectives

After careful study of this chapter, you should be able to:

Discuss the significance of the Past Medical History.

Explain why boundaries between headings may be ignored.

Identify common serious diseases documented in the Past Medical History.

Identify conditions classified as "usual childhood illnesses."

Give examples of questions asked to document an injury.

Differentiate between a true allergy and an abnormal reaction or sensitivity.

Classify statements in the Past Medical History by common subheadings.

For Quick Reference

absence of a limb
actual history
acute illnesses
affirmative answer
alcoholic intoxication
alcoholism
allergic to adhesive tape
allergic to shellfish and peanuts
allergy (pl. allergies)
anaphylactic shock
anemia
arthritis
asthma
blindness
cancer
chronic diseases and disabilities
confinement to bed or wheelchair
continuity
conventionally
conversant
coronary artery disease
criminal violence
diabetes
diabetic
diphtheria
drug addiction
epilepsy
fragment
functional impairments
gastric intolerance
heart attack
heart disease
high blood pressure
historical data
horse dander
hospitalizations
hypertension
immune status
idiosyncratic reaction
immunizations
inadvertent administration of medicine
industrial injuries
injury
kidney disease
known allergies to food or medications
laboratory testing
measles
mental illness
military service
mumps
negatives
nervous or mental disease
paralysis
past episodes
past illnesses
past injuries
perfunctory fashion
photosensitivity

Of the "usual childhood diseases" of a generation ago, only chickenpox now remains usual, the others (measles, mumps, rubella, and whooping cough) having been virtually eliminated by routine immunization of infants and school children. In addition, polio, diphtheria, and rheumatic fever—never so widespread as the other childhood infections but more dangerous—have just about disappeared.

> UCD (usual childhood diseases)

Injuries

To the physician, the terms *injury* and *trauma* suggest a broader range of possibilities than they do to the average lay person. For the purposes of this part of the history, the term is limited to serious injuries such as may result from falls, automobile accidents, industrial injuries, military service, and criminal violence. Examples of injuries that would be included here are fractures, dislocations, severe sprains and strains, open wounds or burns, and any injury that led to scarring or deformity, loss of a body part, or lasting impairment of function. A history of many serious automobile or industrial accidents suggests mental illness, alcoholism, or drug addiction. Patients often conceal or lie about injuries sustained while fighting or engaged in criminal activities.

For both medical and legal reasons, it is customary to assemble as much information as possible about an injury: the exact date, time, and place; physical and anatomic mechanisms of the injury; all attendant circumstances such as poor visibility, bad weather, alcoholic intoxication, or deliberate assault; use of safety devices such seat belts, safety glasses, or guards on machinery; date, place, nature, and outcome of all medical evaluation and treatment, including x-rays and other diagnostic studies, surgery, and physical therapy; and any residual structural or functional impairment. The more remote the injury from the time the history is taken, the less crucial it is to obtain all these details.

Surgical Operations

Even the most minor surgical procedures can result in changes of structure, function, or both that are later mistaken for signs of disease. Patients are seldom conversant with the technical details of their operations, and may even be completely in the dark as to their purposes and effects. They also tend to forget childhood procedures (tonsillectomy, herniorrhaphy) or minor ones (laparoscopy, arthroscopy, vasectomy) when asked point blank about any surgical operations.

> *status post* right inguinal herniorrhaphy

Chronic Diseases and Disabilities

It is understood that material in this section is not considered directly relevant to the problem for which the patient is under evaluation or treatment. Hence chronic conditions such as diabetes, hypertension, rheumatoid arthritis, coronary artery disease, and schizophrenia are more likely to receive mention here than acute illnesses which may well prove to be related to or part of the History of

Present Illness. Significant functional impairments (blindness, paralysis, absence of a limb, confinement to bed or wheelchair) also belong here.

Allergies

Any prior history of allergy or sensitivity, especially to medicines, should be a part of the patient's written records. Usually such information is prominently displayed on the front of a hospital chart or medical office record to prevent inadvertent administration or prescription of a medicine to which the patient has had an untoward response. Besides true allergies, such as violent sneezing due to horse dander and anaphylactic shock precipitated by an injection of penicillin, any abnormal reactions or sensitivities are usually recorded here, such as gastric intolerance to erythromycin and photosensitivity resulting from taking tetracycline. All such are typically lumped together by patients as "allergies" anyway.

> There are no known allergies to foods or medications. Patient may have allergies to pollens and dust.
>
> allergic to penicillin   allergic to bee stings
>
> GI sensitivity to codeine and erythromycin
>
> allergic to adhesive tape
>
> allergic to shellfish and peanuts   idiosyncratic reaction to ibuprofen
>
> She is allergic to penicillin, aspirin, codeine, and does not tolerate Tylenol because of constipation.

Immunizations

Routine childhood immunizations must usually be taken for granted, particularly in an adult, unless written records are available. Military or travel papers may supply dates of immunizations. It is advisable to insert here also any information about the patient's immune status that has been learned through laboratory testing or skin testing.

For Quick Reference

PMH (Past Medical History)
pneumonia
polio
prior history
prior illnesses
recollections
remote history
residuals
resulting current disability
rheumatic fever
rheumatoid arthritis
ROS (Review of Systems)
rubella
scarring or deformity
schizophrenia
sensitivity
sequela (pl. sequelae)
skin testing
stroke
supplemented
surgical operations
surgical treatment
trauma
tuberculosis
UCD (usual childhood diseases)
ulcer
untoward response
usual childhood diseases (UCD)
whooping cough

Exercises for Chapter 6

Review and Summarize

A. Multiple Choice

___ 1. Components of the Past Medical History may include all of the following EXCEPT
   a. Past illnesses.
   b. Past surgeries.
   c. Current medications.
   d. Previous injuries.
   e. Immunizations.

___ 2. Severe adverse reactions to medications as well as environmental irritants and gastric intolerance are included in the discussion of
   a. Past illnesses.
   b. Injuries.
   c. Immunizations.
   d. Current medications.
   e. Allergies.

___ 3. Of the "usual childhood diseases" of a generation ago, which one now remains as the "usual childhood disease"?
   a. Measles.
   b. Mumps.
   c. Whooping cough.
   d. Chickenpox.
   e. Polio.

B. Fill in the Blank

1. The inclusion of information in the Past History implies that it is not _____ to the History of the Present Illness.

2. The Past History may consist largely of _____.

3. The more remote the illness or injury from the time the history is taken, the less _____ it is to obtain full details.

C. Short Answer

1. Why is the surgical history an important factor in elucidating the nature of the current illness?

_____

_____

2. Write a short definition of the following terms. If you can, condense the definition into just a few words or a single synonym that you feel more comfortable with. Note that some words are not medical words. Their application to the medical context may be different from their use in other contexts and may take some extrapolation on your part.

   a. Sequelae _____

   b. Idiosyncratic _____

   c. Perfunctory _____

Pause and Reflect

Do you or someone you know have allergies to food, medications, or other substances? From the author's description of a true allergy versus an abnormal reaction or sensitivity, how would you classify your allergy? What impact might an unreported allergy have on a patient's medical treatment?

_____

_____

_____

_____

_____

_____

Relate and Remember

1. Take a sheet of paper and draw lines to create four columns, labeled A through D. List five important things to remember about the chapter. Put these in column A. In column B, next to each of the items to remember, write the name of an object that might help you to remember the fact. In column C, write the name of a place that might help you to remember the fact. In column D, write a description of a visual image with which you can associate the fact in column A. You may not be able to put something in each column (B through D) for each fact in column A, but don't give up without trying.

2. Create a flow chart or a diagram that illustrates how each part of the Past History relates to the other parts.

Collaborate and Share

Label a blank sheet of paper with your name at the top and write a question requiring a short answer (less than a sentence) related to this chapter. Pass this paper to the student to your right, who will answer the question and then add a question of his or her own, as you answer the question on the paper received from the student on your left. Each sheet moves around the room until everyone has had a turn with every paper and you end up with the paper with your name at the top. Choose the best question(s) and answer(s) from your page to read aloud when called upon by your instructor.

Explain and Learn

Using colored dots (or a drawn dot or star), mark what you feel is the most important point or line in each paragraph of the chapter. If you feel there are multiple important points, rate them and mark the most important with, for example, a red dot, a secondary point with a yellow dot, and the least important point with a green dot. Once you have done this, share your findings with two or three classmates near you. Do you all agree? Discuss any differences of opinion and justify your final decisions.

Relax and Play

1. With another student, role-play doctor-patient, with one of you being the doctor and the other the patient. The doctor questions the patient to obtain a past history using the discussion in this chapter as a guide for questions to ask. The patient may provide truthful answers about his or her own medical history or make up answers; it doesn't matter. After doing this, switch roles and repeat the process. Each of you transcribe the history you obtained as doctor.

2. With students divided into groups, each group selects a different game show ("Who Wants to be a Millionaire," "Jeopardy," "Hollywood Squares," etc.) and creates an "episode" using questions and answers related to this chapter. Select contestants from your game show from other groups. Vote on the best game presented.

Generalize and Apply

Write a statement of something you learned from this chapter and how you think it will help you in your life or career. Crumple the sheet of paper into a "snowball." When the instructor says, "go," toss the "snowball" into the air for other students to catch. When called on by the instructor, read the statement from the snowball you caught to the rest of the class.

Extrapolate and Project

1. Discuss some of the reasons given for incomplete or inaccurate information in the Past History section of the medical report. How critical might these omissions or inaccuracies prove to be? What measures can be taken by both patient and doctor to ensure the greatest accuracy of the past history?

_____

_____

_____

_____

_____

_____

2. Why should healthcare personnel be motivated to keep full and accurate medical records? In what ways and to what extent do you think this responsibility will fall on you in your chosen allied health career?

_____

_____

_____

_____

7

Review of Systems: Head, Eyes, Ears, Nose, Throat, Mouth, Teeth

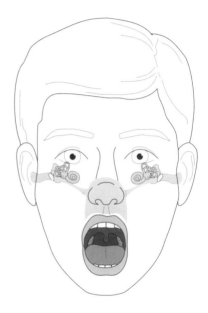

Information recorded in this final section of the Past Medical History, the Review of Systems (not "Review of Symptoms"), is broken down for convenience into an arbitrary classification that does violence to any strictly anatomic or physiologic division of the body into systems. As noted at the beginning of the preceding chapter, the distribution of material in this book has led to a much fuller treatment of historical details under the Review of Systems than would appear in an actual history.

ROS (Review of Systems), System Review

Head

The head is not a system but an anatomic region. In this part of the history the physician records any diseases or injuries of the scalp, skull, and brain and any significant history of headaches. Alternatively, conditions affecting the brain may be taken up in the neurologic history, and disorders of the hair and scalp may be recorded as skin conditions. The organs of special sense (eyes and ears, including balance centers), the upper respiratory tract (nose, sinuses, pharynx), and the mouth and teeth are treated as separate "systems."

Head: No history of headaches or significant head trauma.

Full details of any significant head injury (concussion, skull fracture), no matter how remote in time, are included in the Past Medical History. Of cardinal importance is the establishment of a clear picture of any headache problem, acute or chronic. Headache can be a symptom of life-threatening disease. Moreover, several common types of headache are ordinarily diagnosed on the basis of history alone. In questioning the patient about headaches, the physician seeks to learn their nature, location, frequency, severity, and duration; associated symptoms such as nausea, vomiting, watering of the eye on the affected side, or aching or stiffness in the neck; triggering factors such as fatigue, stress, menstrual periods, hunger, or certain foods; aggravating factors such as coughing, straining, or bending forward; and alleviating factors such as rest, analgesics, or an ice bag. A migraine headache is often preceded by a warning (aura) consisting usually of flashes of light perceived by the patient before the headache begins.

Learning Objectives

After careful study of this chapter, you should be able to:

Describe the organization of the Review of Systems.

Identify conditions and symptoms associated with the head, eyes, ears, nose, mouth, throat, and teeth.

Organize statements from a Review of Systems by category.

Identify information in an HEENT Review of Systems that could be alternatively classified.

For Quick Reference

abnormal taste
absence of taste
ageusia
aggravating factors
airsickness
allergic rhinitis with polyps
allergy shots
alleviating factors
amaurosis fugax
anosmia
astigmatism
aura (warning)
aversion to light
avocational exposure to loud noises
bifocals
bilateral headache
bilateral nasal obstruction
bite plate for TMJ syndrome
bitemporal headache
bitter taste in mouth
black eye
bleeding gums
bleeding in ears
blind spot
bloodshot eyes
bloody nasal mucus
blurring of vision
boring headache
brackish taste in mouth
brain tumor
brassy taste in mouth
bruxism
burr hole
canker sore
carsickness
cataract extraction and lens implant
cautery for nosebleeds
cephalalgia, cephalgia
chapping of lips
clears his throat frequently
clouding of vision
cluster headache
cold sore
color blindness
concussion
congestion
constricting band around the head
copious watery rhinorrhea
corrective lenses or glasses
coryza
crusting of eyelashes
crusting of eyelids
dark bodies in eye
deglutition
dental caries
denture
desensitizing regimen
difficulty of near adaptation

---

scalp laceration requiring sutures

basal, basilar skull fracture

two concussions in childhood, without sequelae

subdural hematoma treated with a burr hole   craniotomy

cephalalgia, cephalgia, headache

headache: bilateral, bitemporal, occipital, frontal, temporal, unilateral

headache: boring, nagging, pounding, splitting, throbbing

"feels like the top of my head is coming off"

headache: nervous, stress, tension   **headache**: histamine, Horton, cluster

headache: hemicrania, migraine, sick   *fortification spectrum*

aura, prodrome, warning   flashes of light, scintillating scotomata

aggravated by any movement of the head, bending forward, coughing, straining

Gives a history of recurrent severe unilateral headaches since childhood, triggered by fatigue or stress, lasting several hours, and associated with nausea, vomiting, and sensitivity to light.

Severe headaches lasting about half an hour occur several times a day and occasionally awaken him at night. The pain seems to be in or behind the right eye and is accompanied by watering and redness of the eye.

A dull nuchal ache radiating into both temples and sometimes feeling like a constricting band around the head.

Eyes

A thorough review of ocular history elicits information about past or present symptoms such as blurring of vision, double vision, partial or complete loss of vision, or difficulty of near adaptation; seeing spots or flashes; seeing halos or rings around lights; undue visual impairment with reduced illumination; pain in, on, or behind the eyeball; redness, discharge, watering, or abnormal sensitivity to light; swelling, drooping, itching, or crusting of lids; and full details about the use of glasses or contact lenses and the date of the most recent eye examination. Eye symptoms can indicate neurologic or systemic rather than purely local disease, as in the case of loss of vision due to a brain tumor or retinopathy due to diabetes.

Eyes: No ocular symptoms or visual deficits.

eyesight, vision, visual acuity

mild uncompensated visual defect   myopia, nearsightedness

blurring, clouding, fogging, fuzziness **of vision**

diplopia, double vision, seeing double   astigmatism

presbyopia, difficulty with near adaptation   farsightedness

diminished peripheral vision, tunnel vision   blind spot, scotoma

amaurosis fugax, transient monocular blindness

sees a curtain, line, shadow in his right eye

sees halos, rings around lights

color blindness   xanthopsia

night blindness, nyctalopia, poor dark adaptation

dark bodies, specks, spots   vitreous floaters

flashes of light, scintillating scotomata, *fortification spectrum*

burning, pain, smarting   **sensation**: foreign-body, gritty, scratchy

pain on blinking   eyestrain

twitching of the right eyelid   drooping, ptosis of the left upper lid

irritation, itching, prickling, soreness, edema, puffiness, swelling **of the eyelid**

bloodshot, red eye   *pinkeye*

photophobia, aversion, sensitivity to light

lacrimation, tearing, watering   crusting, gluing of eyelids

discharge, drainage, matter, mucus, *sand*, *sleep* **in the eye**

crusting, matting of eyelashes

discharge: mucopurulent, stringy, thick, thin, watery

black eye, periorbital ecchymosis, *shiner*

corrective lenses, glasses   reading glasses   safety glasses

contact lenses: disposable, extended-wear, gas-permeable, hard, semisoft, soft

bifocals   trifocals

His most recent eye examination (ophthalmologic examination, refraction) was about 3 years ago.

oculist, ophthalmologist, optician, optometrist

Had bilateral cataract extraction and lens implants about 4 years ago.

Uses Timoptic drops for glaucoma.   wide-angle, narrow-angle glaucoma

Ears

The examiner inquires about the duration, degree, and pitch range of hearing loss in one or both ears; ringing, popping, or other abnormal sounds heard by the patient; pain, pressure, itching, swelling, bleeding, or discharge; history of occupational, avocational, or military exposure to loud noises; history of injury to the ear, particularly perforation of the tympanic membrane; possible effects of air travel or scuba diving on the ears; any ear surgery; and use of a hearing aid. Pain felt in the ear can result from a wide range of non-otic diseases, including pharyngitis, laryngeal cancer, mumps, and brain tumor.

Ears: No history of infection, earache, or hearing loss.

auditory acuity, hearing   deafness, hearing loss, impairment

high-pitch hearing loss   damping, muffling of hearing

acoustic trauma   ototoxic drugs

dysacusis   hyperacusis

wears a hearing aid in the left ear

tinnitus

buzzing, clicking, popping, ringing, roaring, rushing, whistling **in the ear**

earache, otalgia, otodynia   plugged, stopped-up ears

feeling of pressure, stuffiness   draining, *gathering, running ears*

bleeding, discharge, drainage, draining, oozing, running, seeping **from the ear**

itching, swelling   otorrhea

For Quick Reference

difficulty swallowing
diminished peripheral vision
diplopia
dizziness, dizzy
double vision
drainage in the eye
dried blood in nasal secretions
drooling
drooping of upper eyelid
dryness of mouth
dysequilibrium
dysgeusia
dysphagia lusoria
dysphonia
ear plugs
edema of eyelid
effects of air travel on the ears
effects of scuba diving on the ears
epistaxis treated with silver nitrate
    cautery and anterior packs
exposure to dust or tobacco smoke
extended-wear contact lenses
eyestrain
false teeth
farsightedness
fatigue
fever blister
flashes of light before headache
fogging of vision
foreign-body sensation
fortification spectrum
foul taste in mouth
frequency of headache
frequent colds
frequent sneezing
"frog in the throat"
frontal headache
frontal sinus pain and pressure
fullness in periorbital regions
fuzziness of vision
gagging
gas-permeable contact lenses
giddiness
glaucoma
globus hystericus
globus sensation
gluing of eyelids
gritty sensation
halos (rings around lights)
hard contact lenses
hay fever
headache triggered by fatigue or stress
hearing loss
hearing protection at work
hemicrania
histamine headache
hoarseness
Horton headache

For Quick Reference

> swimmer's ear, otitis externa, *"fungus"*
> scuba diving   perforated, ruptured tympanic membrane
> PE (poly, polyethylene tubes)   wears ear plugs, hearing protection at work
> mastoiditis, mastoidectomy

Vertigo and **dysequilibrium**, suggesting disease of the inner ear, are usually dealt with here also. The distinction between these two symptoms is sometimes difficult to make; lay persons refer to both as "dizziness." Vertigo is a constant or intermittent feeling that one is spinning ("like I just got off a merry-go-round"). In contrast, dysequilibrium means difficulty maintaining one's balance when standing or walking. Vertigo is usually accompanied by some degree of dysequilibrium, but dysequilibrium often occurs alone. Several drugs can produce temporary impairment of hearing or balance, and a history of their use may be significant.

> dizziness, dysequilibrium, imbalance, unsteadiness
> Ménière disease, syndrome
> motion sickness, carsickness, seasickness, airsickness
> giddiness, spinning, swimming sensation, vertigo
> dizzy, off balance, unbalanced, unsteady, wobbly

Nose

The nasal history includes mention of any acute or chronic pain, swelling, obstruction, or discharge affecting the nose; sneezing, nosebleeds, or frequent colds; seasonal or occasional allergies; sinus infections; disturbance of the sense of smell; history of fracture or other injuries; submucous resection for deviated septum, removal of polyps, cautery for nosebleeds, or other surgical procedure; and regular or long-term use of decongestants or antihistamines for nasal symptoms, particularly inhalers, drops, or sprays. The common cold is a universal human experience. Members of the laity often apply the generic term *cold* or *sinus* (*trouble*) to any condition characterized by nasal obstruction and discharge. Hence careful and detailed questioning may be needed to elicit clues to nasal allergy, chronic irritation from dust or smoke, or obstruction due to a tumor. The lay meaning of congestion usually diverges from the correct technical sense, "swelling due to engorgement of blood vessels."

> Nose: Denies frequent colds, epistaxis, or nasal fracture.
> No history of trauma, obstruction, nosebleed, or discharge.
> irritation, itching, pain, prickling, soreness, tingling **of the nose (nares)**
> nasal blockage, congestion, obstruction, pressure, stuffiness
> He has to blow his nose constantly.
> URI (upper respiratory infection)
> nasal congestion provoked by recumbency, alcohol consumption, and changes
>   in temperature and humidity
> coryza, nasal discharge, rhinorrhea, runny nose, sniffles

copious watery rhinorrhea   bloody nasal mucus

thick yellowish-green discharge   dried blood in the nasal secretions

sneezing, sternutation

sneezing: frequent, paroxysmal, repeated, repetitive, staccato

violent sneezing spells triggered by exposure to dust or tobacco smoke

She has clear nasal discharge, sneezing, and itching of the nasal mucous membranes, worse when around cats or dust.

bloody nose, epistaxis, nasal hemorrhage, nosebleed

chronic allergic rhinitis with polyps   vasomotor rhinitis

hay fever, rose fever, seasonal rhinitis   perennial rhinitis

The patient has a 4-day history of purulent rhinorrhea, bilateral nasal obstruction, and a sensation of fullness in the periorbital regions.

frontal sinus pain and pressure for several days

anosmia   undisplaced fracture of the nasal bones

recurrent epistaxis in the past treated with silver nitrate cautery and anterior packs

long-term, chronic   use, abuse   of nose drops, sprays

underwent a submucous resection for deviated septum

allergy shots, desensitizing regimen, hyposensitization, immunotherapy

Throat

The throat includes not only the pharynx, the common channel shared by the respiratory and digestive tracts, but also the larynx. Important historical points include sore throat (the most common presenting symptom in many outpatient practices), postnasal drip, choking, and difficulty swallowing; atypical throat pain, which may be due to foreign body, abscess, tumor, or neurologic disease; hoarseness or other change in the voice; and history of tonsillectomy or other

Throat: Denies sore throat, hoarseness, or difficulty swallowing.

Has frequent bouts of tonsillitis which cause him to miss work and require antibiotic treatment.

needs to clear his throat frequently   mucus, phlegm

postnasal drainage, discharge, drip, catarrh   choking, gagging

throat: sore, scratchy, raw, irritated, swollen, inflamed

pharyngitis   strep throat

deglutition, swallowing

dysphagia, difficulty in swallowing, pain on swallowing

globus hystericus, globus sensation, lump in the throat

dysphagia lusoria

can hardly swallow his own saliva

Sore throat is worse in the morning and evening but very mild or absent during the day.

hoarseness, dysphonia, *"frog in the throat"*

T&A (tonsillectomy and adenoidectomy) in childhood

For Quick Reference

phlegm
photophobia
pink toothbrush
pinkeye
poor dark adaptation of eyes
popping of ears
postnasal catarrh
postnasal discharge
postnasal drainage
postnasal drip
pounding headache
presbyopia
pressure in ears
prickling of eyelid
prickling of nose
prodrome
profuse salivation
ptosis of upper eyelid
ptyalism
puffiness of eyelid
purulent rhinorrhea
raw throat
reading glasses
red eye
refraction
remote in time
removal of polyps
repeated or repetitive sneezing
retinopathy due to diabetes
rhinorrhea
ringing of ears
ROS (Review of Systems)
rose fever
rotten taste in mouth
runny nose
ruptured tympanic membrane
safety glasses
saline taste in mouth
salty taste in mouth
sand in the eye
scalp laceration
scintillating scotomata
scotoma (pl. scotomata)
scratchy sensation
scratchy throat
seasickness
seasonal or occasional allergies
seasonal rhinitis
seeing double
sees halos or rings around lights
sees spots or flashes
semisoft contact lenses
sequela (pl. sequelae)
severity of headache
shiner
sialorrhea
sick headache
significant head trauma

For Quick Reference

throat operation. Pain, swelling, or mass in the neck is included here for convenience.

Mouth and Teeth

These are not the exclusive province of the dentist. The oral and dental history can have important health implications. Chronic, painful conditions of the mouth, gums, or teeth can severely impair nutrition. Many systemic diseases are reflected in oral and dental symptoms. A recent history of dental work may provide a clue to bacteremia with ensuing infective endocarditis. The complete oral and dental history includes soreness, swelling, or ulceration of the lips, gums, or tongue; excessive salivation or excessive dryness of the mouth; abnormal taste or absence of taste; bleeding gums; frequent toothache or sensitivity of teeth to sweet, hot, or cold food or drinks; dental caries; loose, damaged, or missing teeth; regularity of dental care; and wearing of orthodontic braces, dentures, or other appliances.

burning, chapping, rawness, soreness, stinging, swelling **of the lips**

cold sore, fever blister   canker sore

taste (in the mouth): bitter, brackish, brassy, foul, metallic, rotten, saline, salty, sour

ageusia, food has no taste   dysgeusia

dryness of the mouth, tongue, throat   xerostomia

excessive, profuse salivation, ptyalism, sialorrhea   drooling

bleeding, sensitivity, soreness, swelling, ulceration **of the gums**

pink toothbrush

tickling of the palate

burning, irritation, rawness, soreness **of the tongue**

chewing, mastication   bruxism, tooth-grinding

frequent toothaches

denture, false teeth   partial, bridge, plate

orthodontic braces, retainer

wears a bite plate prescribed by an oral surgeon for TMJ syndrome

Exercises for Chapter 7

Review and Summarize

A. Multiple Choice

___1. Conditions affecting the brain may be covered under the heading "HEENT" in the Review of Systems OR under which of the following:
a. Cardiovascular.
b. Respiratory.
c. Musculoskeletal.
d. Neurologic.
e. Circulatory.

___2. Disorders of the hair and scalp may be recorded under the heading "HEENT" in the Review of Systems or under which of the following headings:
a. Musculoskeletal.
b. Neurologic.
c. Dermatologic.
d. Circulatory.
e. Allergies.

___3. The most frequent condition explored related to the head is
a. Skull fracture.
b. Subdural hematoma.
c. Seborrhea and psoriasis.
d. Headache.
e. Brain tumor.

___4. Pain in the ear may be an indication of non-otic diseases such as
a. Brain tumor.
b. Allergies.
c. Colds.
d. Influenza.
e. Circulatory problems.

___5. The symptom patients describe as "dizziness" may be either dysequilibrium or
a. Otalgia.
b. Otodynia.
c. Otorrhea.
d. Vertigo.
e. Aura.

B. Fill in the Blank

1. The mouth and teeth are not the exclusive province of the dentist because many _____

   are reflected in oral and dental symptoms.

2. The establishment of a clear picture of any acute or chronic headache problems is of _____

   importance.

3. Eye symptoms may indicate a neurologic problem such as a _____ or a systemic

   problem such as _____ .

4. Disease of the inner ear may be suggested by the symptoms of _____ or

   _____ .

C. Short Answer

Write a short definition of the following terms. If you can, condense the definition into just a few words or a single synonym that you feel more comfortable with.

1. Aura_____

2. Cardinal (importance)_____

3. Fortification spectrum_____

4. Prodrome_____

5. Amaurosis fugax_____

6. Xanthopsia _____

7. Nyctalopia_____

8. Vertigo_____

9. Coryza_____

10. Deglutition_____

11. Xerostomia_____

12. Bruxism_____

Pause and Reflect

In discussing both the Past Medical History and now the Review of Systems, the author suggests that the actual recording of these two parts of the complete history may be much more condensed and brief than his discussion implies. What do you think is the reason for this? Do you think it's important to be as thorough as the text discussion every time a patient is seen or admitted to the hospital? Is a thorough review of these two parts of the history important for every illness or disease with which a patient might present? How might the Past History and Review of Systems be tailored to the specific circumstance?

_____

_____

_____

_____

_____

_____

Relate and Remember

Using this outline of the head, list 3 to 5 terms (you may use the terms in the shaded boxes) for each part or area that the physician might use to describe the symptoms experienced by a patient in the HEENT Review of Systems.

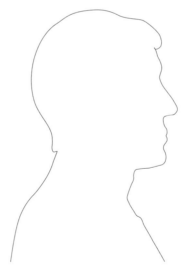

Collaborate and Share

On a 3" x 5" card, write a question pertaining to the chapter. The instructor will collect the cards and divide the class into small groups. Each group gets a portion of the questions to answer and share with the class.

Explain and Learn

1. Turn to the person next to you (or behind or in front of you), and share with each other one important piece of information you got from this chapter. Also share how you might use this information in your life or in your work. If you have a question that wasn't answered in the chapter, share that as well. If your partner doesn't have the answer, ask your instructor.

2. In groups of 3 to 5 students, list on a sheet of paper everything you know about this chapter. The group then picks 1 to 3 most important points to share with the class.

Relax and Play

1. In small groups, create a mind map. On a piece of poster board, large piece of butcher paper, or a brown paper grocery bag opened up and spread flat, draw a circle in the center. From the circle draw lines at the end of which are other circles. A third level can be added if desired. In the main circle, place a word or phrase that represents the main point of the chapter. In the secondary or tertiary circles, put words or phrases that represent additional important points. With the members of the group standing around the mind map, take turns tossing a coin onto the map. The person tossing the coin explains the term on which the coin landed (or nearest term). Continue until each term is discussed or until instructor calls "time."

2. Select 10 to 20 words or phrases from the word list in this chapter and create a word search puzzle. Rather than list the words you've chosen, however, list the definitions as clues. Copy the puzzles to share with the rest of the class. Students must first determine which word goes with the definition before finding it in the puzzle.

Generalize and Apply

In discussing the Head, Eyes, Ears, Nose and Throat portion of the Review of Systems, the author points out that symptoms in these areas may indicate illness or disease in other areas. Summarize in writing the systemic problems mentioned in the text that may be reflected in the HEENT review. Can you think of any conditions the author didn't mention that might also be reflected in this review? In transcribing a report, how might knowing about these illnesses be helpful to you?

_____

_____

_____

_____

Compare and Contrast

Compare the nose, ears, eyes, throat, or mouth and teeth (choose only one) and the things that can go wrong with them to objects in your environment (plants, rocks, machines, furniture, buildings, etc.). How are they alike? How are they different?

_____

_____

_____

_____

_____

_____

Extrapolate and Project

You are probably beginning to see how difficult it can be for physicians to come up with a diagnosis when symptoms in the eyes, for example, can be an indication of diabetes. Speculate on how the physician might begin to narrow down the list of possibilities. Keep this in mind as you continue studying this textbook.

_____

_____

_____

_____

_____

_____

_____

_____

_____

_____

8

Review of Systems: Cardiovascular

The cardiovascular system includes the heart with its covering membrane, the pericardium, and all the blood vessels of the body—arteries, arterioles, capillaries, venules, and veins. Disorders of this system can produce a remarkable diversity of symptoms, from cough to ankle swelling and from sudden blindness to sudden death.

> Cardiovascular: Denies chest pain, palpitation, dyspnea, orthopnea, PND, intermittent claudication, and history of rheumatic fever, heart murmur, hypertension, or heart attack.

Patients' complaints with respect to the cardiovascular system can be divided into three groups: those rightly perceived as related to the heart or blood vessels, such as angina pectoris, an irregular pulse, or varicose veins; those due to heart or blood vessel disease but not so perceived by the patient, such as anorexia, orthopnea, and ankle edema due to congestive heart failure; and those wrongly attributed by the patient to cardiovascular disorders, such as chest pain actually due to indigestion or tingling in the extremities falsely blamed on "poor circulation."

The cardiovascular history begins with a review of past diagnoses of congenital or acquired heart murmurs, rheumatic fever, enlarged heart, coronary artery disease, heart attack, high blood pressure, varicose veins, thrombophlebitis, and treatments, past or present, prescribed for any of these. Note is made of the results of past diagnostic studies such as electrocardiograms, echocardiograms, stress testing, cardiac catheterization, and angiography, and of any surgical procedures, such as pacemaker implantation, valve repair or replacement, and coronary artery bypass graft.

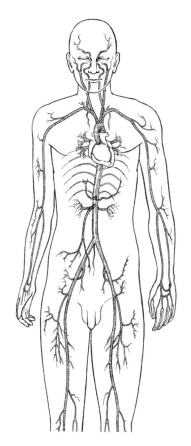

Learning Objectives

After careful study of this chapter, you should be able to:

Define the scope of the cardiovascular system.

Describe the cardiovascular history-taking process.

Identify complaints related to the cardiovascular system.

Classify cardiovascular conditions by major diagnostic categories.

Name common cardiovascular diagnostic studies and procedures.

> He was told he had a cardiac murmur of unknown type in high school.
> Had MI's 5 and 2 years ago with uneventful recoveries.
> Barlow syndrome, mitral valve prolapse with regurgitation
> cardiac catheterization
> functional, innocent heart murmur   echocardiogram
> stress test, treadmill test   ECG, EKG (electrocardiogram)
> coronary angiogram, arteriogram
> phlebogram, venogram, Doppler ultrasound study
> WPW (Wolff-Parkinson-White) syndrome   PAT (paroxysmal atrial tachycardia)
> CABG (coronary artery bypass graft)   valvulotomy

For Quick Reference

acquired heart murmur
angina at rest
angina decubitus
angina pectoris
angiography
ankle edema
anorexia
arterial embolism
arteriolar disease
arteriole
artery
atypical angina
Barlow syndrome
breathlessness
CABG (coronary artery bypass graft)
calf claudication
calf cramps
capillary
cardiac catheterization
claudication
coldness and pallor in fingers
congenital heart murmur
congestive heart failure
coronary angiogram or arteriogram
coronary arteriosclerosis
coronary artery disease
cramping in the calf
crushing chest pain
CVA (cerebrovascular accident)
delirium
dementia
dependent edema
dermatitis with pigmentation or
   ulceration
diffuse arteriolar spasm
dilated varicose veins
diversity of symptoms
DOE (dyspnea on exertion)
Doppler ultrasound study
drawing feeling in the calf
dyspnea
dyspnea at rest
ECG, EKG (electrocardiogram)
echocardiogram
enlarged heart
exertional dyspnea
flip-flop in the chest
flopping in the chest
fluttering in the chest
functional heart murmur
heart attack
heart murmur
heaviness in the calf
heaviness in the chest
high blood pressure
hip claudication
hypertension
innocent heart murmur

The physician tends to bracket cardiovascular disorders according to six or seven well-defined diagnostic categories: coronary arteriosclerosis, valvular heart disease, and hypertension, any of which can lead to the group of syndromes called congestive heart failure; pericardial disease; local or generalized arteriosclerosis; and venous disease (varicose veins, phlebitis, thromboembolism).

Because coronary artery disease is a major cause of disability and death, any complaint of **chest pain** must be carefully evaluated to determine whether it represents angina pectoris, the cardinal symptom of coronary disease. The historical elaboration on a complaint of chest pain has been set forth at length in Chapter 1 and will not be reviewed in detail here. A full description of chest pain includes its character, intensity, location, extent, radiation, duration, and frequency of occurrence; the effect of position, movement, breathing, and swallowing; associated symptoms such as shortness of breath, sweating, and cardiac palpitation; the effect of resting or taking medicines such as antacids or nitroglycerin; and triggering factors such as physical exertion, smoking, eating, strong emotion, or exposure to cold.

> heaviness, pain, pressure, weight on (in) the chest
>
> angina pectoris   angina decubitus   atypical, unstable, variant angina
>
> angina at rest   Prinzmetal angina
>
> recurring episodes of intense, diffuse, crushing chest pain radiating into the neck, jaw, left shoulder, and left arm. Attacks of pain are precipitated by exertion or emotional upset, sometimes by a heavy meal, and relieved by rest and sublingual nitroglycerin.

When shortness of breath is due to **cardiac failure** it is typically less oppressive in the upright position (orthopnea) and may occur in attacks that awaken the patient during the night (paroxysmal nocturnal dyspnea, PND). Orthopnea is graded by the number of pillows needed to avoid respiratory distress. Wheezing, coughing, and exertional dyspnea are common to cardiac and noncardiac disorders. Ankle swelling is a frequent early symptom of cardiac failure but also occurs in other conditions, one of which will be mentioned shortly. Typically the swelling is worst at the end of the day and resolves partly or completely overnight.

> dyspnea, shortness of breath (SOB), breathlessness, short-windedness, respiratory distress
>
> dyspnea at rest   DOE (dyspnea on exertion), exertional dyspnea
>
> PND (paroxysmal nocturnal dyspnea)   3-pillow orthopnea
>
> ankle, dependent, pedal edema

The term **palpitation** can indicate unduly forceful heartbeat, unduly rapid heartbeat, irregular heartbeat, or simply an abnormal awareness of one's heartbeat. Even the most skilled interviewer may occasionally fail to determine just which of these the patient has experienced. Of cardinal importance regarding palpitation are the frequency and duration of attacks; associated symptoms such as light-headedness, weakness, shortness of breath, or chest pain; and triggering factors such as exertion, eating, smoking, or use of certain medicines.

> flip-flop, flopping, fluttering, palpitations, pounding, thumping in the chest
> missing, skipping a beat   conscious of his heartbeat at night
> paroxysmal tachycardia

Peripheral arteriosclerosis causes symptoms by impairing the blood supply to critical organs such as the brain and kidney or to the extremities. Hence the symptoms vary according to the structures affected. **Cerebrovascular disease** can lead to a wide variety of symptoms, including headaches, light-headedness, confusion, drowsiness, sensory or motor impairment, behavioral disorders, delirium, dementia, seizures, transient ischemic attacks, and stroke. These symptoms will usually be considered in the neurologic and psychiatric portions of the history.

> TIA (transient ischemic attack)
> CVA (cerebrovascular accident), stroke

Narrowing of a major artery supplying blood to an extremity can cause muscle cramps, weakness, coldness, pallor, and numbness. Intermittent **claudication** (from Latin *claudicare* "to limp") is the classical symptom of circulatory impairment in the lower extremity. The patient describes intense, disabling cramping in the calf, less often in the foot, shin, or thigh, which comes on with walking and is promptly relieved by rest. Similar symptoms can affect the upper extremity after exertion. Intermittent claudication can be graded according to the distance (e.g., 1 mile, 2 flights of stairs, 3 city blocks) that the patient can walk without symptoms. When vascular obstruction occurs in the distal aorta or common iliac artery, the male patient may experience impotence as well as intermittent claudication (Leriche syndrome).

> intermittent claudication   hip, thigh, calf claudication
> can walk about 4 blocks before pain begins
> Calf cramps come on after he has walked about one-half mile and require him to
>   stop and rest.

Coldness, pallor, numbness, and pain in an extremity can also be caused by sudden obstruction of the arterial supply by a traveling clot (arterial embolism), by arteriolar disease, or by diffuse arteriolar spasm (Raynaud phenomenon). Hence the duration, extent, severity, and intermittency of these symptoms must be carefully ascertained.

> Raynaud phenomenon
> She occasionally has spells of extreme coldness and pallor in 3 fingers of the left
>   hand, especially after going outdoors in cold weather.

For Quick Reference

intermittent claudication
irregular heartbeat
irregular pulse
leaking veins
Leriche syndrome
light-headedness
local or generalized arteriosclerosis
MI (myocardial infarction)
missing a beat
mitral valve prolapse with
   regurgitation
motor impairment
muscle aching
orthopnea
pacemaker implantation
pain in the chest
painless edema
pallor of extremity
palpitation of heart
palpitations in the chest
paroxysmal tachycardia
PAT (paroxysmal atrial tachycardia)
pedal edema
pericardial disease
peripheral arteriosclerosis
phlebitis
phlebogram
PND (paroxysmal nocturnal dyspnea)
poor circulation
pounding in the chest
predisposing factors
pressure in the chest
Prinzmetal angina
prolonged standing
Raynaud phenomenon
respiratory distress
rheumatic fever
seizures
sensory impairment
shortness of breath
short-windedness
skipping a beat
SOB (shortness of breath)
stress testing
stroke
sublingual nitroglycerin
thigh claudication
3-pillow orthopnea
thromboembolism
thrombophlebitis
thumping in the chest
TIA (transient ischemic attack)
tingling in the extremities
tortuous varicose veins
transient ischemic attacks
traveling clot
treadmill test
triggering factors

For Quick Reference

Varicose veins are dilated, tortuous, sometimes leaking veins, usually in the lower extremities. The condition is common and familial. It can be mild and cause no symptoms other than unsightly bulging of superficial veins, but some persons with varicosities experience ankle swelling, muscle aching, and dermatitis with pigmentation or ulceration.

> varices, varicosities, varicose veins
>
> Has had swollen veins in both legs above and below the knees for about 10 years. These are asymptomatic except for a rare drawing feeling or heaviness in the left calf after prolonged standing.

Thrombophlebitis is the formation of an obstructing clot within the lumen of an inflamed vein. Local injury, oral contraceptives, and sudden immobilization by illness, injury, or surgery are predisposing factors. Thrombophlebitis in a deep vein can cause edema and aching of the extremity, but is often asymptomatic. **Deep venous thrombosis** can result in sudden release of a clot into the circulation, with lethal consequences (pulmonary embolism). For this reason, any complaint of peripheral swelling will prompt a thorough inquiry into its duration, severity, and intermittency, and the presence of any predisposing factors for thrombophlebitis.

> Noted gradual onset of painless edema in the left foot, ankle, and calf during the past 72 hours.

Exercises for Chapter 8

Review and Summarize

A. Multiple Choice

___ 1. Cardiovascular complaints can be divided roughly into three groups which include all the following EXCEPT
    a. Those perceived to be benign.
    b. Those perceived correctly as related to heart or blood vessels.
    c. Those due to the heart but not perceived as such.
    d. Those incorrectly perceived to be due to the heart.

___ 2. Diagnostic categories into which cardiovascular disorders can be divided include all of the following EXCEPT
    a. Coronary arteriosclerosis.
    b. Pericardial disease.
    c. Thrombophlebitis.
    d. Venous disease.
    e. Local or generalized arteriosclerosis.

___ 3. Peripheral arteriosclerosis involving the cerebral vascular system is likely to be covered under which of these Review of Systems headings?
    a. Cardiovascular.
    b. Head, Eyes, Ears, Nose and Throat.
    c. Musculoskeletal.
    d. Neurologic.
    e. Genitourinary.

___ 4. Peripheral vascular disease is often mistakenly thought to apply only to the circulatory problems in the extremities but may apply as well to the (Mark two)
    a. Coronary arteries.
    b. Kidneys.
    c. Heart valves.
    d. Cerebrovascular system.
    e. Deep veins of the lower extremities.

___ 5. Any of the following might be designated palpitation EXCEPT
    a. Abnormally slow heartbeat.
    b. Unusually forceful heartbeat.
    c. Unusually rapid heartbeat.
    d. Irregular heartbeat.
    e. Abnormal awareness of heartbeat.

B. Fill in the Blank

1. Chest pain due to indigestion may be attributed by the patient to _____.

2. Shortness of breath due to cardiac failure is usually less severe in the _____ position.

3. Orthopnea is usually graded by how many _____ are needed to avoid respiratory distress.

4. The symptoms of peripheral arteriosclerosis vary according to the _____ affected.

5. Disabling cramping in the calf due to circulatory impairment is referred to as _____

   _____.

6. Coronary arteriosclerosis, valvular heart disease, and hypertension can each lead to _____

   _____ .

C. Short Answer

1. List the main diagnostic categories given in the text for heart disease.

   _____

   _____

   _____

   _____

   _____

   _____

2. List the parameters that are included in a full description of chest pain.

   _____

   _____

   _____

   _____

   _____

   _____

3. How is claudication graded?

    _____

4. Why will any complaint of peripheral swelling prompt a thorough inquiry by the physician?

    _____

    _____

5. Write a short definition of the following terms. If you can, condense the definition into just a few words or a single synonym that you feel more comfortable with.

    a. Orthopnea _____

    b. Claudication _____

    c. Innocent (heart murmur) _____

    d. Dyspnea _____

Pause and Reflect

1. Using different colored highlighters or crayons, underline or highlight important points or main ideas of the chapter. Circle key words. Use symbols (such as stars, asterisks, exclamation point, question mark, etc.) meaningful to you to mark key words and phrases. Summarize the information you thought most important from the chapter. If you had any questions, write those out to share with classmates or to ask your instructor.

    _____

    _____

    _____

    _____

    _____

    _____

    _____

    _____

2. Draw a mind map to illustrate the various categories of cardiovascular diseases and the symptoms that accompany them.

Relate and Remember

1. Refer to the explanation for a metaphor in the review questions for Chapter 1. Think of a metaphor that completes this statement: The human heart is like a _____. Use a visual or a verbal metaphor. You may fill in the blank with the name of an object or draw (or cut out of a magazine) a picture representing one or more important points. Explain your choice.

_____

_____

_____

_____

_____

_____

_____

_____

2. Using this outline of the human body, list 3 to 5 terms for each area that the physician might use to describe the cardiovascular symptoms experienced by a patient in that area.

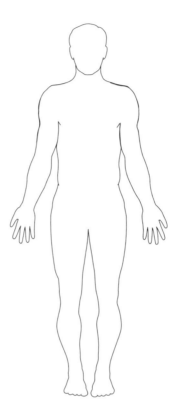

Collaborate and Share

After every student has read the chapter, divide into groups of 3 to 5. Divide the chapter so that each group has a portion. Re-read your section. As a group, write questions based on your section. They may be multiple choice, short answer, or fill in the blank. The number of questions will depend on how large a section of the chapter your group is covering, but will probably only be two or three at most. You may even ask the same question in different ways. A spokesperson for each group may then ask the rest of the class its questions or the instructor can collect them and compile them to be distributed to each student.

Explain and Learn

1. Working in pairs, take turns pointing out and explaining the important points or main idea of each paragraph or section.

2. Type on a separate sheet or handwrite below a sample Cardiovascular Review of Systems for a patient with some form of heart disease. Use as many of the terms in the shaded boxes as appropriate. Explain why you included certain points. Remember to include both positives and negatives.

_____

_____

_____

_____

_____

_____

Relax and Play

1. On a 3" x 5" card, write a question pertaining to the chapter and give it to your instructor. The instructor, using a koosh ball, small stuffed animal, net bath sponge, or some other soft object, asks the question, then tosses the object at random to an individual student who answers the question.

2. Fold a blank piece of paper in half three times so that when unfolded there are eight squares. Write one thing you learned in each square. Move around the room, asking other students to define or explain an item on your sheet. That student then signs the square. The student who gets all eight squares signed first wins.

Generalize and Apply

Write on a 3" x 5" card a statement of something you learned and how you think this information will help you or a question as yet unanswered. Turn in this card to the instructor as your "ticket out" of class.

Compare and Contrast

1. What is the difference between *varicose veins* and *thrombophlebitis*?

_____

_____

_____

2. Compare the heart and the things that can go wrong with it to objects in your environment (plants, rocks, furniture, buildings, etc.). How are they alike? How are they different?

_____

_____

_____

_____

_____

Extrapolate and Project

Since chest pain can be an indication of diseases other than heart disease, such as gastric ulcer, musculoskeletal pain, or pulmonary disease, which do you think should be ruled out first? Why? What might be the consequences of failing to rule out heart disease before exploring other causes of chest pain?

_____

_____

_____

_____

_____

_____

_____

_____

_____

_____

_____

9

Review of Systems: Respiratory

Properly speaking, the respiratory system includes all bodily structures concerned with the handling of air: the nose and paranasal sinuses; the mouth and pharynx; the larynx and trachea; the lungs with their bronchi, bronchioles, alveoli, and terminal air sacs; the pleura; and the chest wall and diaphragm with their nerve supplies. However, the parts of this system other than the tracheobronchial tract and the lungs are usually dealt with in other parts of the Review of Systems.

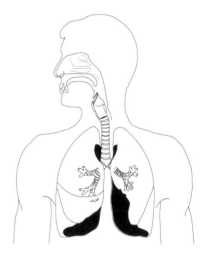

> Respiratory: No history of asthma, bronchitis, pneumonia, chronic cough, hemoptysis, or purulent sputum.

The respiratory history begins with a survey of past or current diagnoses of respiratory problems such as asthma, bronchitis, pneumonia, emphysema, pleurisy, pneumothorax, tuberculosis, and lung cancer, with treatments prescribed for any of these. Lay persons often misunderstand the terms *asthma* and *bronchitis* and apply them indiscriminately and inappropriately to various pulmonary and nonpulmonary complaints. The subject is questioned about shortness of breath (intermittency, severity, inciting factors), cough, and chest pain. As noted in the preceding chapter, these three symptoms can also indicate cardiac disease. Dyspnea is a cardinal feature of asthma. Generally there is audible wheezing as well, and cough, which may produce thick sputum.

> asthma, asthmatic bronchitis, bronchial asthma, RAD (reversible airways disease)
>
> pulmonary emphysema, COPD (chronic obstructive pulmonary disease)
>
> chronic bronchitis   bronchiectasis
>
> pneumonia, pneumonitis
>
> dyspnea, shortness of breath (SOB), breathlessness, short-windedness, respiratory distress
>
> a feeling of not being able to draw a full breath
>
> congestion, heaviness, pain, pressure, tightness **in the chest**
>
> rawness in the chest, bronchial irritation

The significant features of a cough are its frequency and severity, factors that provoke it (such as cold air, smoke, dust, or lying down), and the character and volume of sputum produced. Hemoptysis (coughing up blood) demands careful investigation because it can indicate pulmonary malignancy, pulmonary infarction, or, less often, tuberculosis. Often the subject cannot reliably distinguish between

Learning Objectives

After careful study of this chapter, you should be able to:

Name the structures included in the Respiratory Review of Systems.

Describe common respiratory symptoms and conditions.

Identify terminology related to the respiratory system.

Classify statements as belonging to a Respiratory Review of Systems.

For Quick Reference

asthmatic bronchitis
audible wheezing
blood-streaked sputum
bloody sputum
brassy cough
bronchial asthma
bronchiectasis
bronchitis
bubbling cough
COPD (chronic obstructive pulmonary
 disease)
coughing up blood
croupy cough
dyspnea
emphysema
expectorated material
foul-tasting sputum
frothy sputum
gelatinous sputum
hacking cough
hemoptysis
hollow cough
inciting factors
irritation of the pleura
loose cough
metallic cough
mucous
mucus
nasopharyngeal secretions
paroxysmal wheezing
phlegm
pleurisy
pleuritic pain
pneumonitis
pneumothorax
productive cough
pulmonary emphysema
pulmonary infarction
pulmonary malignancy
purulent sputum
putrid sputum
RAD (reversible airways disease)
rasping cough
rattling cough
respiratory allergies to pollen, molds,
 and dust
respiratory distress
ropy sputum
rusty sputum
short-windedness
SOB (shortness of breath)
spitting (up) blood
stitch
tracheobronchial tract
tuberculosis
viscid or viscous sputum
watery sputum
wracking cough

expectorated material (brought up from the trachea or lungs) and nasopharyngeal secretions.

> Exercise brings on attacks of paroxysmal wheezing and coughing, dyspnea, and production of clear, viscous sputum.
>
> **cough**: brassy, bubbling, croupy, hacking, harsh, hollow, loose, metallic, nonproductive, productive, rasping, rattling, wracking
>
> cough productive of purulent sputum   mucus, phlegm, sputum
>
> brings up, coughs out, coughs up, expectorates, expels, raises
>
> **sputum**: blood-streaked, foul-tasting, frothy, gelatinous, green, purulent, putrid, ropy, rusty, viscid, viscous, watery, yellow
>
> bloody sputum, coughing (up) blood, hemoptysis, spitting (up) blood

Sharply localized, stabbing pain in the chest that is aggravated by taking a deep breath and virtually abolished by breathholding is called *pleuritic* because it typically results from irritation of the pleura (the membrane lining the thoracic cavity and covering the lungs) due to pleurisy, pneumonia, pulmonary infarction, or chest wall injury. The lungs themselves contain no pain-sensitive nerves.

> catch, pleuritic pain, *stitch*

If the smoking history and details of any known respiratory allergies have not previously been recorded, they may be brought in here.

> Patient is a 44-pack-year cigarette smoker with mild respiratory allergies to pollen, molds, and dust.

Exercises for Chapter 9

Review and Summarize

A. Multiple Choice

____ 1. Sharply localized, stabbing chest pain aggravated by deep breathing and relieved by breathholding may be due to
   a. Heart attack.
   b. Pulmonary embolism.
   c. Pleurisy.
   d. Musculoskeletal chest pain.
   e. Costochondritis.

____ 2. Respiratory distress includes all of the following EXCEPT
   a. Dyspnea.
   b. Shortness of breath.
   c. Hemoptysis.
   d. Breathlessness.
   e. Short-windedness.

B. Fill in the Blank

1. Although the respiratory system, strictly speaking, involves all the structures involved in air handling, only the

   _____ and the _____ are covered under the Respiratory Review of Systems.

2. Patients apply the terms _____ and _____ indiscriminately and inappropriately to a

   number of pulmonary and nonpulmonary complaints.

3. A patient often cannot reliably distinguish between _____ and nasopharyngeal secretions.

4. The lungs themselves contain no _____ nerves.

C. Short Answer

   Write a short definition of the following terms. If you can, condense the definition into just a few words or a single synonym that you feel more comfortable with.

1. Asthma_____

2. Bronchitis_____

3. Hemoptysis_____

Relate and Remember

Using this outline of the trachea, bronchi, and lungs, list 3 to 5 symptoms and several differential diagnoses for each that the physician might consider when conducting a respiratory review of systems.

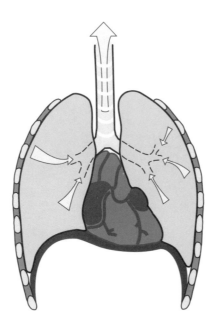

Collaborate and Share

On a paper bag, write your name and the statement, "I want to know more about . . ." Pass the bag around the room. The other students write what they know about the question on a piece of paper and initial their answers, placing the paper inside the bag. When your bag returns to you, summarize the information in the bag. Share the summaries with the class.

Explain and Learn

In groups of 3 to 5, with each group assigned a different section of the chapter, discuss and agree on the important points or main ideas. Put them into your own words. Select one person to present your summary to the class.

Relax and Play

1. On a 3" x 5" card, write a question pertaining to the chapter and give your card to the instructor, who then asks the class the questions. The student with the answer "pops up" to answer the question. If the student answers correctly, the instructor tosses the student a "fun-size" candy bar.

2. With another student, role-play doctor-patient. The doctor elicits a Respiratory Review of Systems from the patient for a complaint or disease of the patient's choosing. Be sure to consider both positive and negative responses. After doing this, switch roles and using different complaints/disease, repeat the process. Type a Respiratory Review of Systems based on the responses you received as doctor.

Compare and Contrast

Compare the respiratory system and the things that can go wrong with it to objects in your environment (plants, rocks, machines, furniture, buildings, etc.). How are they alike? How are they different?

_____

_____

_____

_____

Extrapolate and Project

What three symptoms might be an indication of either pulmonary disease or heart disease? How can it be determined whether these three symptoms relate to heart disease or pulmonary disease? What types of pulmonary disease or heart disease might cause chest pain? What are the differences in character of the chest pain when pulmonary in origin or cardiac in origin? (Remember the parameters used to define chest pain as discussed in Chapter 1 and Chapter 8. You may need to go outside the text to get a complete answer to these questions.)

_____

_____

_____

_____

_____

_____

_____

_____

_____

10

Review of Systems: Gastrointestinal

The digestive system, like the respiratory system, begins at the lips. However, symptoms affecting the mouth, teeth, tongue, salivary glands, and throat are usually considered in other parts of the history. The gastrointestinal history is concerned mainly with two types of symptoms: abdominal pain of any type or degree (though abdominal pain often results from nondigestive causes) and any disturbances of digestive function, including anorexia, nausea, vomiting, and diarrhea. Symptoms due to disorders of the liver or biliary tract, the pancreas, or the rectum or anus are also included here.

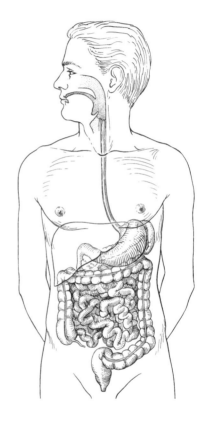

> GI: No history of nausea, vomiting, diarrhea, constipation, abdominal pain, weight loss, or melena.
>
> Denies fatty food intolerance, jaundice, vomiting, or any past history of GI disease.

In reviewing the past digestive tract history, the examiner inquires about previous diagnoses of hiatal hernia, ulcer, gallstones or gallbladder disease, pancreatitis, or colitis; any tumors of the alimentary canal or associated structures; results of endoscopic studies (esophagoscopy, gastroscopy, colonoscopy), gastrointestinal x-rays, or other diagnostic studies; operations on the digestive organs, including appendectomy and hemorrhoid surgery; and use of antacids, laxatives, enemas, or prescription medicines for digestive symptoms. Because lay persons often diagnose their own conditions as gas, ulcers, or indigestion, the physician must exercise caution in accepting such diagnoses.

> peptic ulcer disease   cholecystitis with cholelithiasis
> inflammatory bowel disease   Crohn disease, regional enteritis
> pancreatitis   *tic*   diverticulum   ulcerative colitis
> Upper GI showed hiatal hernia with gastroesophageal reflux.
> A *Helicobacter pylori* antibody study performed last April was negative.
> Barium enema showed colonic diverticulosis with diverticulitis.
> Sonogram of the gallbladder was negative for stones.
> had a *bleed*, GI hemorrhage   Mallory-Weiss syndrome
> bleeding esophageal varices   bowel obstruction
> appendectomy   cholecystectomy   laparoscopy
> colostomy   ileostomy   exploratory laparotomy   lysis of adhesions

Learning Objectives

After careful study of this chapter, you should be able to:

Name the structures included in a Gastrointestinal (GI) Review of Systems.

Describe common GI complaints and conditions.

Name common diagnostic tests and studies of the GI system.

Identify terminology related to the GI system.

Classify statements as belonging to the GI Review of Systems.

For Quick Reference

A full description of abdominal pain runs along much the same lines as a description of chest pain. The interviewer elicits exact information about the location, radiation, character, severity, and intermittency of abdominal pain, any aggravating or mitigating factors, and, in particular, relation to diet and to digestive and eliminative functions.

> epigastric, substernal distress   burning, heartburn, pyrosis
>
> colicky, crampy, intermittent pain   cardiospasm
>
> bloating, flatulence, gas, gassiness, heaviness, oppression, stuffiness
>
> constant severe pain in the epigastrium, radiating to the back between the scapulae and relieved by sitting up or lying on the right side
>
> intolerance to eggs, cucumbers, onions, and apples

Abdominal pain may be described as burning, crampy, or dull. It may be constant, intermittent, or of varying intensity. It may remain in one place or radiate or migrate to another, perhaps in the back or chest. It may be brought on, aggravated, or relieved by eating, not eating, drinking, having a bowel movement, or assuming certain positions. It may be provoked by taking certain medicines, eating certain foods; a record of any food intolerances is an important part of the digestive history.

Symptoms besides abdominal pain that draw attention to the digestive system are anorexia, nausea, pain or difficulty in swallowing that seems to originate below the pharynx, vomiting, flatulence (excessive intestinal gas), constipation, diarrhea, abnormal appearance of the stools, weight loss, jaundice, and anorectal pain, swelling, or bleeding. A history of vomiting prompts inquiries about its frequency and the volume and character of emesis. Blood mixed with gastric contents often has a characteristic coffee-grounds appearance. Jaundice, a yellow color of the skin, mucous membranes, and ocular sclerae, indicates an excessive quantity of bile pigment in blood and tissues. It can result from intrinsic liver disease (hepatitis, hepatic failure) or from obstruction of the biliary tract by a gallstone or a tumor.

> anorexia, loss of appetite, poor appetite
>
> early satiety, setophobia
>
> bulimia, polyphagia   pica
>
> nauseated, nauseous, queasy, sick at her stomach, upset stomach
>
> *"butterflies in the stomach"*
>
> dysphagia   difficulty, pain on swallowing
>
> vomit, throw up, regurgitate, experience emesis
>
> gag, retch, choke   *dry heaves*   *water brash*
>
> postprandial nausea and vomiting   morning sickness   emesis, vomitus
>
> **emesis**: bilious, bloody, bright red, coffee-grounds
>
> flatulence, flatus, gas, passing gas, wind
>
> borborygmus, growling, gurgling, rumbling
>
> aerophagia   hiccups, singultus
>
> (acid) eructations, belching, burping   "food repeats on me"
>
> icterus, jaundice

Because constipation and diarrhea mean different things to different people, the interviewer must carefully determine the frequency and consistency of the patient's stools. Even with normal **bowel habits**, an abnormal stool color can indicate disease. Clay-colored stools occur in obstruction of the biliary tract because bile does not reach the intestine. Blood that has passed through much of the intestine before appearing in the stool may look tarry black (melena) because of chemical changes in blood pigment caused by digestive enzymes. When the patient reports bleeding with bowel movements, the interviewer inquires whether the blood was seen only on the toilet paper or was on the surface of the stool or mixed with it. Mucus, pus, undigested food, and parasites such as tapeworms are other possible abnormal findings in the stool. Complaints of anal pain, itching, swelling, or protrusion are also part of the digestive history.

BM (bowel movement), defecation, elimination, feces, stools

Bowel habits are regular.

Has daily BM's with 2 to 3 episodes of constipation a month, for which he takes MOM.

Stools have been dark but not tarry.

Stools have been soft, formed, and easy to pass.

stools: acholic, black, bloody, bulky, clay-colored, floating, formed, foul-smelling, hard, liquid, loose, mushy, pale, *rabbit, ribbon*, runny, tarry, watery

constipation, irregularity, obstipation   tenesmus

diarrhea, loose stools, runs   lientery

encopresis   steatorrhea

hematochezia   melena

blood, mucus, pus mixed with stools

blood in the toilet bowl, noted only on the toilet paper

cathartic, laxative, physic

dyschezia, painful defecation   straining at stool

anal itching, anal pruritus, pruritus ani   proctalgia fugax

hemorrhoids, piles   anal bulging, mass, protrusion

fecal incontinence, leakage, soiling

Weight loss is a usual consequence of anorexia but it can also indicate severe systemic disease, grossly inadequate diet, or malabsorption. If the subject's dietary history has not been reviewed earlier, it may be brought in here, as well as the use of coffee, alcohol, tobacco, and other substances known to affect digestive function.

Inguinal hernia may also be considered with the gastrointestinal history because most hernias contain loops of bowel and eventually affect digestive or eliminative function. The subject is asked about swelling or bulging in the groin or scrotum that is accentuated by coughing or straining and diminishes or disappears in the recumbent position.

bulging, fullness, protrusion, swelling **in the groin**

burning, stinging sensation in the left groin on coughing, straining at stool, or lifting heavy loads

For Quick Reference

gastroesophageal reflux
gastroscopy
GERD (gastroesophageal reflux disease)
GI (gastrointestinal) hemorrhage
heartburn
heaviness
Helicobacter pylori antibody study
hematochezia
hemorrhoidectomy
hemorrhoids
hepatic failure
hepatitis
hernia
hiatal hernia
hiccups (hiccoughs)
ileostomy
incontinence
inflammatory bowel disease
jaundice
laparoscopy
lientery
lysis of adhesions
malabsorption
Mallory-Weiss syndrome
melena
mitigating factors
MOM (milk of magnesia)
nausea
obstipation
pancreatitis
passing gas
peptic ulcer disease
pica
piles
polyphagia
postprandial nausea and vomiting
proctalgia fugax
protrusion in the groin
pruritus ani
pyrosis
regional enteritis
regurgitate
scapulae
setophobia
singultus
sonogram of gallbladder
steatorrhea
straining at stool
stuffiness
substernal distress
tarry black stools
tenesmus
tic
ulcer
ulcerative colitis
vomiting
water brash
weight loss

Exercises for Chapter 10

Review and Summarize

A. Multiple Choice

____ 1. The adjective that describe a fluid wave in the abdomen is
   a. Ascetic.
   b. Acidic.
   c. Asthenic.
   d. Ascitic.

____ 2. Postprandial pain is experienced after
   a. Waking.
   b. Sleeping.
   c. Eating.
   d. Belching.

____ 3. The movement that propels food from the esophagus to the stomach is termed (Mark two.)
   a. Peristalsis.
   b. Deglutition.
   c. Absorption.
   d. Digestion.

____ 4. In a patient with a bleeding peptic ulcer, one would expect the patient's stools to be
   a. Streaked with bright red blood.
   b. Clay-colored.
   c. Black.
   d. Chalky.

B. Fill in the Blank

1. Like the respiratory system, the GI system begins at the _____.

2. A record of _____ intolerances is an important part of the digestive history.

3. Excessive intestinal gas is known as _____.

4. Jaundice indicates an excessive quantity of _____ in blood and tissues.

C. Short Answer

1. What are the two types of symptoms primarily covered in the gastrointestinal review of systems? What else is covered?

_____

_____

_____

_____

2. Why is it necessary for the physician to carefully explore complaints of diarrhea or constipation? What kinds of questions might one ask to elucidate whether a patient has either of these problems?

_____

_____

_____

_____

_____

_____

3. Write a short definition of the following terms. If you can, condense the definition into just a few words or a single synonym that you feel more comfortable with.

a. Hematemesis _____

b. Melena _____

c. Polyphagia _____

d. Pica_____

e. Borborygmus_____

f. Singultus_____

Relate and Remember

Take a sheet of paper and draw lines to create four columns, labeled A through D. List five important things to remember about the chapter. Put these in column A. In column B, next to each of the items to remember, write the name of an object that might help you to remember the fact. In column C, write the name of a place that might help you to remember the fact. In column D, write a description of a visual image with which you can associate the fact in column A.

Collaborate and Share

In small groups, draw a mind map on a piece of poster board, a large piece of butcher paper, or a brown paper grocery bag opened up and spread flat. With the members of the group standing around the mind map, take turns tossing a coin onto the map. The person tossing the coin explains the term on which the coin landed (or nearest term). Continue until each term is discussed or until instructor calls "time."

Explain and Learn

Using colored dots (or a drawn dot or star), mark what you feel is the most important point or line in each paragraph. If you feel there are multiple important points, rate them and mark the most important with, for example, a red dot, a secondary point with a yellow dot, and the least important point with a green dot. Once you have done this, share your findings with two or three classmates near you. Do you all agree? Discuss any differences of opinion and justify your final decisions.

Relax and Play

1. Select 5 to 10 words or phrases from the terms included in this chapter. Write a poem or song that incorporates these terms in such a way as to reveal their meaning or use. If writing a song, use a familiar tune or rap style.

2. Select 10 to 20 words or phrases from the word list in this chapter and create a word search puzzle. Rather than list the words you've chosen, however, list the definitions as clues. Copy the puzzles to share with the rest of the class. Students must first determine which word goes with the definition before finding it in the puzzle.

Generalize and Apply

1. What information is sought by the physician when reviewing past digestive tract history? Why must the physician exercise caution in accepting a patient's own diagnosis?

    _____

    _____

    _____

    _____

    _____

    _____

2. What information is sought concerning the characteristics of abdominal pain? How does differentiating the nature of the pain relate to arriving at a differential diagnosis? Give examples.

    _____

    _____

    _____

    _____

    _____

Compare and Contrast

Compare the gastrointestinal tract and the things that can go wrong with it to objects in your environment (plants, machines, rocks, furniture, buildings, etc.). How are they alike? How are they different?

    _____

    _____

    _____

    _____

    _____

Extrapolate and Project

As with all the Review of Systems, the actual time spent elucidating the patient's history and current complaints as well as the extent to which this information is recorded in the medical report varies based on the relevance it has to the presenting complaint. When might an extensive review and record of the GI system be relevant? What conditions of other systems might require the ruling out of specific GI complaints?

_____

_____

_____

_____

_____

_____

_____

_____

_____

_____

_____

11

Review of Systems: Genitourinary

The kidneys and urinary tract (ureters, bladder, and urethra) and the reproductive system are considered together because of their close anatomic association and the frequency with which both organ systems are affected simultaneously by disease. A thorough review of genitourinary (GU) history includes past diagnoses of congenital anomalies of the urinary or genital tract; urinary tract infections; stone in a kidney, ureter, or bladder; sexually transmitted diseases; genitourinary surgery; and menstrual and reproductive history.

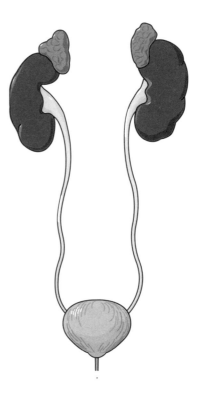

UTI (urinary tract infection)   GU (genitourinary)

cystitis   acute, chronic glomerulonephritis

pyelonephritis   nephrotic syndrome

calculus, gravel, stone, urolithiasis   stone-former

horseshoe kidney   polycystic kidney

IVP (intravenous pyelogram) showed a bifid ureter on the left.

renal function   vesicoureteral reflux

cystoscopy   circumcision

hysterectomy   BSO (bilateral salpingo-oophorectomy)

oophorectomy   vasectomy

tubal ligation   prostatectomy

DES daughter   *Chlamydia*   bacterial vaginosis

STD (sexually transmitted disease)   *clap*, GC (gonorrhea)

Candida, yeast

PID (pelvic inflammatory disease)

Other significant history is a laparotomy $2^1/_2$ years ago, at which time multicystic ovaries with thickened capsules were observed.

Lay persons often erroneously attribute back pain to kidney disease and often assume that any urinary tract infection involves the kidneys. Hence the interviewer must be wary of accepting patients' statements about the kidneys. Symptoms suggesting renal or urinary tract disease are pain in one or both flanks, increase in frequency of urination (as opposed to increase in urine volume), nocturia (being awakened at night by the urge to void), burning or pain on voiding, difficulty voiding, diminution in the urinary stream, incontinence of urine, bedwetting in an older child or adult, blood in the urine, and any other marked change in the appearance of the urine.

Learning Objectives

After careful study of this chapter, you should be able to:

Name the structures of the genitourinary (GU) and reproductive systems.

Describe common symptoms and diagnoses associated with the GU and reproductive systems.

Identify terminology related to the kidneys and urinary tract.

Explain the methods by which the female reproductive history is recorded.

Classify statements as belonging to the Genitourinary Review of Systems.

For Quick Reference

back, CVA (costovertebral angle), flank pain

making water, micturition, passing water, passing urine, urination, voiding

pollakiuria, frequency   urgency   hesitancy   dribbling

polyuria   oliguria   anuria   hematuria   double voiding

urine: bloody, cloudy, Coca-Cola, concentrated, dark, smoky

incontinence: dribbling, drip, overflow, stress, urge

nocturia times 3   dysuria, burning on urination, painful urination

catheterized   Foley, indwelling, urethral catheter

The **menstrual history** includes age at onset of menses (menarche), regularity of cycles, interval between periods, duration of periods, and the date of the last normal menstrual period. In addition, the interviewer inquires about menstrual cramps (dysmenorrhea), heaviness of flow, and intermenstrual or postmenopausal bleeding.

Menstrual: Menarche occurred at age 11. Periods are regular with an interval of 29 days and a 4- to 5-day flow.

catamenia, menses, (menstrual) periods

LMP (last menstrual period)   *flooding*   *spotting*

passing clots and tissue   cramps, dysmenorrhea

PMS (premenstrual syndrome)   mittelschmerz, ovulatory pain

change of life, climacteric, menopause   hot flashes, flushes

surgical menopause   primary, secondary amenorrhea

oligomenorrhea   polymenorrhea   hypermenorrhea   menorrhagia/metrorrhagia

pubarche   thelarche

The **female reproductive history** covers pregnancies, miscarriages, abortions, stillbirths, normal deliveries, and cesarean births; and any complications of pregnancy such as hemorrhage or toxemia. In recording the reproductive history,

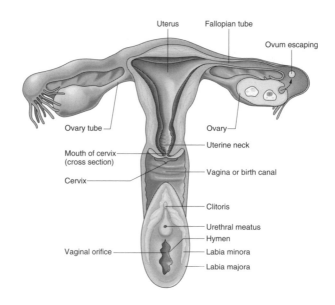

physicians use a kind of shorthand in which the term *gravida* (abbreviated G) refers to pregnancies and *para* (abbreviated P) to their outcome. Thus "gravida 3, para 3" refers to a woman who has been pregnant three times and has delivered three children. A more elaborate notation uses four numerals after "para," denoting respectively full-term deliveries, preterm deliveries, miscarriages or abortions, and living children. This recording system sometimes proves ambiguous with respect to multiple pregnancies (twins, triplets) and their outcome.

parity   *gravida 3, para 3, ab 1*

primigravida   nulligravida   primipara   multipara

genital lesion, ulcer, wart   pruritus vulvae

discharge: creamy, curdy, foul-smelling, frothy, thick, thin, watery, white, yellow

hyperemesis   eclampsia, preeclampsia, toxemia of pregnancy

C-section (cesarean section)

Women are also questioned about the use of condoms, diaphragms, oral contraceptives, or other contraceptive methods; pelvic pain, vaginal discharge, vulvar itching, sores, or rash; and any breast complaints (pain, swelling, masses, bleeding or discharge from the nipple).

cystic mastitis, fibrocystic disease of the breast

bleeding, discharge from the nipple   nursing   lactation

Examines her own breasts once a month and has noted no masses or tenderness.

OC (oral contraceptive), birth control pill, the pill   morning-after pill

condom, diaphragm, foam, jelly, spermicidal

coitus interruptus, onanism, withdrawal

Men are questioned about urethral discharge or burning; itching, rash, ulcers, nodules, or other lesions of the genitals; pain or swelling in the testicles; scrotal masses; and infertility.

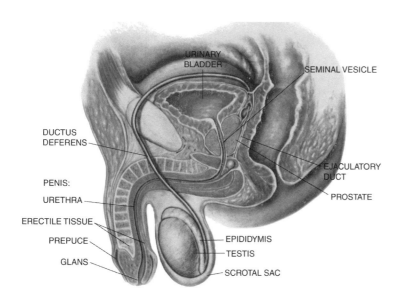

DUCTUS DEFERENS

PENIS:

URETHRA

ERECTILE TISSUE

PREPUCE

GLANS

URINARY BLADDER

SEMINAL VESICLE

EJACULATORY DUCT

PROSTATE

EPIDIDYMIS

TESTIS

SCROTAL SAC

For Quick Reference

G (gravida)
GC (gonorrhea)
genital lesion
genital ulcer
genital wart
glomerulonephritis
GU (genitourinary)
hematuria
hemorrhage
homosexual
horseshoe kidney
hot flashes and flushes
hyperemesis
hypermenorrhea
hysterectomy
impotence
incest
incontinence of urine
increase in urine volume
indwelling catheter
infertility
intermenstrual bleeding
IVP (intravenous pyelogram)
kidneys and urinary tract
lactation
laparotomy
lesbian
LMP (last menstrual period)
maintaining erection
masturbation
menarche
menopause
menorrhagia/metrorrhagia
menses
menstrual history
micturition
miscarriages
mittelschmerz
morning-after pill
multicystic ovaries
multipara
multiple pregnancies (twins, triplets)
nephrotic syndrome
nocturia
nulligravida
OC (oral contraceptive)
oligomenorrhea
oliguria
onanism
oophorectomy
oral contraceptive
oral sex
orgasm
overflow incontinence
ovulatory pain
P (para)
painful urination
paramour

For Quick Reference

parity
passing clots and tissue
pederasty
pedophilia
PID (pelvic inflammatory disease)
PMS (premenstrual syndrome)
pollakiuria
polycystic kidney
polymenorrhea
polyuria
postmenopausal bleeding
preeclampsia
premature ejaculation
preterm deliveries
primary amenorrhea
primigravida
primipara
prostatectomy
pruritus vulvae
pubarche
pyelonephritis
renal function
reproductive system
scrotal mass
secondary amenorrhea
sexual partner
sexual preference
sodomy
spermicidal
spotting
stable monogamous relationship
STD (sexually transmitted disease)
still births
stone-former
stone in a kidney, ureter, or bladder
stress incontinence
surgical menopause
testicular pain
testicular swelling
thelarche
toxemia of pregnancy
tubal ligation
urethral burning
ureters, bladder, and urethra
urethral catheter
urethral discharge
urge incontinence
urinary tract infection
urolithiasis
UTI (urinary tract infection)
vaginal discharge
vasectomy
vesicoureteral reflux
voiding
voyeurism
vulvar itching
yeast

chancre, *haircut*	genital lesion, ulcer, wart
urethral discharge	

Most persons are reticent about sexual matters, and not much is gained by determined probing unless the chief complaint involves the reproductive system in some way. When necessary, the interviewer may ask about the subject's sexual preference, frequency of sexual activity, number of different partners, participation in oral or anal sex, masturbation, and satisfaction with sexual activity. In addition, men are asked about difficulty in achieving or maintaining erections and premature or delayed ejaculation, women about pain during intercourse and any difficulty in attaining orgasm.

coitus, (sexual) intercourse, sex	climax, orgasm	
anorgasmia, frigidity	dyspareunia	
diminished libido		
erectile dysfunction, impotence	inability to get, maintain, sustain an erection	
gay, homosexual, lesbian		
consort, lover, paramour, (sexual) partner		
stable monogamous relationship		
frottage	masturbation	
anal intercourse, anal sex, sodomy	cunnilingus	fellatio
voyeurism	exhibitionism	pedophilia, pederasty
fetishism	incest	

Exercises for Chapter 11

Review and Summarize

A. Multiple Choice

___ 1. Which condition is NOT a symptom of renal or urinary tract disease?
   a. Oliguria.
   b. Nocturia.
   c. Dysuria.
   d. Hematuria.
   e. Dysmenorrhea.

___ 2. All of the terms below mean "to pass urine" EXCEPT
   a. Void.
   b. Urinate.
   c. Masticate.
   d. Micturate.

___ 3. The term *urolithiasis* literally means
   a. Ureteral stone.
   b. Kidney stone.
   c. Renal stone.
   d. Urine stone.

B. Fill in the Blank

1. The genitourinary review includes history of abnormalities and complaints related to the _____,

   _____, and _____ tracts.

2. The genital tract covers all the organs of the _____ system.

3. The urinary tract covers the _____, _____, and _____.

4. Being awakened at night by the urge to void is called _____.

5. _____ is a word meaning the onset of menses.

C. Short Answer

1. What is included in a thorough review of the genitourinary history?

   _____

2. What symptoms might be reviewed in discussing the urinary tract?

   _____

3. What history is included in the female reproductive history?

   _____

4. What symptoms are reviewed in discussing the female genital tract?

   _____

5. What symptoms are reviewed in discussing the male genital tract?

   _____

6. Write a short definition of the following terms. If you can, condense the definition into just a few words or a single synonym that you feel more comfortable with.

   a. Micturition _____

   b. Congenital anomaly _____

   c. Urolithiasis_____

   d. Pollakiuria _____

   e. Enuresis _____

   f. Oliguria _____

   g. Anuria _____

   h. Catamenia _____

   i. Climacteric_____

   j. Thelarche _____

   k. Onanism _____

Pause and Reflect

Draw a mind map for this chapter using the genitourinary system as the center and the genital and reproductive tracts as two primary components. To these add the historical and symptomatic points discussed in the chapter.

Relate and Remember

1. Answer the following question: The genital tract is like a _____. Use a visual or a verbal metaphor. You may fill in the blank with the name of an object or draw (or cut out of a magazine) a picture representing one or more important points. Explain your choice in light of the information given in this chapter.

_____

_____

_____

_____

_____

_____

_____

2. Compare the reproductive tract (you may choose male or female or both) and the things that can go wrong with it to objects in your environment (plants, machines, rocks, furniture, buildings, etc.). How are they alike? How are they different?

_____

_____

_____

_____

Collaborate and Share

Share your mind map with others in your group. After discussing any disagreements on what should go where, draw a larger map that can be placed on the floor. With all members of the group standing around the map, take turns tossing a coin onto the map and explaining the term or phrase on which the coin lands.

Explain and Learn

1. Explain the difference between *oliguria, anuria, polyuria*, and *pollakiuria*.

_____

_____

_____

_____

2. Explain the difference between *frequency, urgency*, and *enuresis*.

_____

_____

_____

Relax and Play

1. With another student, role-play doctor-patient. With one of you being the doctor and the other the patient, elicit a genitourinary review. Be sure to explore historical information and any current complaints, remembering that both positives and negatives are important. After doing this, switch roles and using different complaints/disease, repeat the process. Transcribe the information you elicited as doctor.

2. Select 10 to 20 words or phrases from the word list in this chapter and create a word search puzzle. Rather than list the words you've chosen, however, list the definitions as clues. Copy the puzzles to share with the rest of the class. Students must first determine which word goes with the definition before finding it in the puzzle.

Compare and Contrast

In what ways does the genital review differ between men and women? In what ways is it similar?

_____

_____

_____

_____

Extrapolate and Project

Considering the prevalence of sexually transmitted diseases today, discuss in writing (or with one or more people and summarize in writing) the necessity for a reliable sexual history. Why is this so difficult to obtain? What can be done to garner a more accurate report? Why might this information be important (or if it's not, why not) when the patient has no genitourinary or sexual problems?

_____

_____

_____

_____

_____

_____

_____

_____

_____

12

Review of Systems: Neuromuscular

This broad category includes disorders of the central and peripheral nervous systems and injuries and diseases that affect not only skeletal muscle but also bones, joints, ligaments, and associated structures. The subject is questioned about prior diagnosis of, and treatment for, seizures, brain concussion, brain tumor, stroke, paralysis, neuritis, any fractures or dislocations, severe sprains, bursitis, tendinitis, or arthritis.

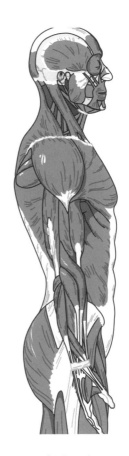

Neuromuscular: There is no history of syncope, seizures, peripheral neuropathy, fractures, dislocations, back pain, or arthritis.

arthritis, arthralgia, arthropathy, rheumatism   lumbago   sciatica

bursitis   tendinitis   lateral epicondylitis, tennis elbow

carpal tunnel syndrome

HNP (herniated nucleus pulposus), ruptured intervertebral disk, slipped disk

calf cramps, night cramps   metatarsalgia   fibromyalgia

DJD (degenerative joint disease), osteoarthritis   ankylosing spondylitis

There is a remote and poorly documented history of rheumatoid arthritis, but she has been free of joint symptoms for at least 5 years.

convulsive disorder, epilepsy, seizure disorder

Symptoms suggestive of **central nervous system disease** are severe or unusual headache; unexplained drowsiness or dysequilibrium; confusion; disorientation; sudden deterioration of memory, judgment, or emotional stability; tremors; incoordination; disorders of speech; weakness, clumsiness, paralysis, or spasticity of the extremities; and seizures. Often, detailed information on these points must be obtained from someone other than the patient. In obtaining a full picture of any of these symptoms, the interviewer asks whether it is constant, intermittent, or progressive; to what extent it impairs normal function; and whether any cause can be suggested for the symptom, such as a recent or remote injury or use of alcohol or drugs.

blackout, fainting, *falling out,* loss of consciousness, passing out, syncope

dopey, draggy, drowsy, lethargic, sluggish, somnolent, woozy   hypersomnia

dizzy, giddy, lightheaded   dysequilibrium, vertigo

confusion, delirium   aphasia

TIA (transient ischemic attack)   RIND (reversible ischemic neurologic deficit)

Learning Objectives

After careful study of this chapter, you should be able to:

Define the scope of the Neuromuscular Review of Systems.

Name symptoms of central nervous system disease.

Describe common diagnoses involving the central nervous system.

Identify terminology associated with the central and peripheral nervous systems, back, and extremities.

Construct a Neuromuscular Review of Systems.

For Quick Reference

absence seizure
anesthesia
ankylosing spondylitis
arm goes to sleep
arthralgia
arthritis
arthropathy
baby the injured part
back pain
barked
brain concussion
brain tumor
bursitis
calf cramps
carpal tunnel syndrome
causalgia
CNS (central nervous system)
convulsion
convulsive disorder
convulsive episode
dead feeling
dislocation
DJD (degenerative joint disease)
drop attack
epilepsy
favor the injured part
febrile seizure
fibromyalgia syndrome
fit
formication
fracture
game
gimpy
gout
grand mal seizure
heavy feeling
HNP (herniated nucleus pulposus)
hobble
hyperesthesia
hypesthesia, hypoesthesia
jacksonian epilepsy
jacksonian march
jacksonian seizure
jammed
jerked
lame
lateral epicondylitis
limp
lumbago
luxation
major motor seizure
meralgia (paresthetica)
metatarsalgia
migratory polyarthralgia
neuritis
night cramps
numbness
osteoarthritis

CVA (cerebrovascular accident), stroke, brain attack
activity level, activity status   bedfast, bedridden
self care   ADL's (activities of daily living)   *toileting*

In gathering data about **syncopal episodes** or seizures, the physician will try to learn from an observer whether the patient displayed any warning signs of distress, cried out, fell, lost consciousness completely or only became confused; whether there was local or general twitching or writhing of the extremities; whether the patient was incontinent of urine during the seizure; and how long after the seizure any weakness, drowsiness, or confusion remained.

convulsion, convulsive episode, fit, seizure, spell
absence, petit mal   drop attack, spell
grand mal, major motor seizure   febrile, jacksonian, uncinate seizure
jacksonian epilepsy   *jacksonian march*

Peripheral nerve disorders are suggested by numbness, paresthesia (a tingling or "pins and needles" sensation), weakness, or paralysis in an extremity. The pain of peripheral neuritis is often described as stinging or burning and often seems to shoot along or just under the surface like an electric shock. The diagnostician inquires whether symptoms are brought on or aggravated by fatigue, certain activities or positions, or a cold or damp environment, and whether there has been exposure to toxic drugs or chemicals.

anesthesia, hyp(o)esthesia, hyperesthesia, paresthesia
numbness, heavy, dead feeling   arm goes to sleep
formication, pins and needles, prickling, tingling
shocklike sensations shooting from the elbow down to the wrist
burning, causalgia, stinging   meralgia (paresthetica)
vague aches and pains all over

Most painful, inflammatory **conditions of the back and extremities** are due to injury—either a single violent event or repeated strains or overuse. Hence the interviewer will attempt to elicit a history of trauma or unusual activities (moving furniture, sudden excessive athletic activity, change of job). Less likely possibilities are local infection and systemic or chronic disorders such as rheumatoid arthritis, fibromyalgia syndrome, and gout. As with pain anywhere, an effort is made to establish a complete profile of back or extremity pain by learning its exact location, radiation, severity, intermittency, aggravating or mitigating factors, and effect on normal function. A patient complaining of muscle or joint pain will be asked about concomitant heat, swelling, stiffness, or spasm, and the effects of rest, exercise, and medicines.

fracture, broken bone   dislocation, luxation   subluxation

sprain, strain   jammed, *stoved*, stubbed   *barked*, scraped, skinned

jerked, sprained, strained, twisted, wrenched

game, *gimpy*, lame, *trick*   limp, hobble

baby, favor the injured part

arthralgia, arthritis, arthropathy   migratory polyarthralgia

myalgia   *crick* in the neck

cramp, drawing, pulling, spasm   *charley horse, shin splints*

backache, back pain, dorsalgia, lumbago

nuchal aching, spasm, tenseness, tightness

arthroscopy   meniscectomy   diskectomy, laminectomy

open reduction and internal fixation   hip pinning

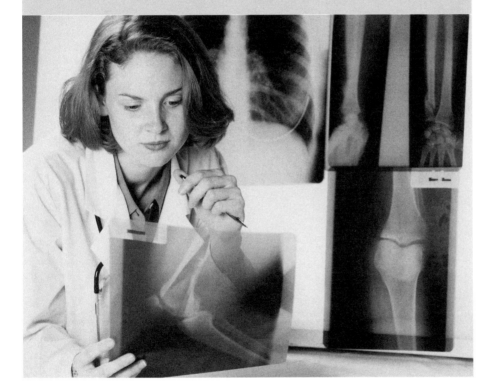

For Quick Reference

paralysis
paresthesia
peripheral nerve disorder
peripheral neuritis
peripheral neuropathy
petit mal seizure
"pins and needles" sensation
prickling
rheumatism
rheumatoid arthritis
ruptured intervertebral disk
sciatica
scraped
seizure disorder
shocklike sensations
skinned
slipped disk
spell
sprain
sprained
stinging
stoved
strain
strained
stroke
stubbed
subluxation
syncopal episode
syncope
tendinitis
tennis elbow
tingling
trick
twisted
twitching of the extremities
uncinate seizure
wrenched
writhing of the extremities

Exercises for Chapter 12

Review and Summarize

A. Multiple Choice

___ 1. Which one of the following choices describes *peripheral neuritis*?
  a. A stinging or burning sensation.
  b. Twitching of the extremity.
  c. Mottled appearance of the overlying skin.
  d. Generalized confusion.

___ 2. A patient with a neuromuscular disorder would likely be asked about prior treatment for
  a. A sexually transmitted disease.
  b. Episodes of severe shortness of breath.
  c. Sudden, rapid heartbeat.
  d. Fractures or dislocations.

___ 3. Most painful or inflammatory conditions of the back and extremities are caused by
  a. The aging process.
  b. Trauma.
  c. Prolonged use of medication.
  d. Tumors.

B. Fill in the Blank

1. A tingling or "pins and needles" sensation is known as _____.

2. The nervous system is categorized into the _____ and _____

nervous systems.

C. Short Answer

1. List the symptoms suggestive of central nervous system disease.

_____

_____

_____

_____

_____

2. Write a short definition of the following terms. If you can, condense the definition into just a few words or a single synonym that you feel more comfortable with.

a. Incoordination _____

b. Intermittent _____

c. Remote_____

d. Dysequilibrium _____

e. Syncope _____

f. Elicit _____

g. Mitigating _____

h. Uncinate_____

3. A physician ascertains if certain symptoms were present before, during, or after a seizure. List these symptoms.

_____

_____

_____

_____

_____

Pause and Reflect

Read this chapter aloud, by yourself or taking turns with other students. If you don't know the meaning or pronunciation of a word, look it up. As you read, pause and reflect on key points at the end of each section. Make notes in the margins of your book, mark with dots or stars, and draw lines from key ideas to subordinate points. Summarize your reading in outline form below.

_____

_____

_____

_____

_____

Relate and Remember

1. Think of a metaphor that completes this statement: The neuromuscular system is like a _____ _____. Use a visual or a verbal metaphor. You may fill in the blank with the name of an object or draw (or cut out of a magazine) a picture representing one or more important points. Explain your choice.

_____

_____

_____

_____

_____

2. Using this outline of the human body, list 3 to 5 terms for each area that the physician might use to describe the neuromuscular symptoms experienced by a patient in that area.

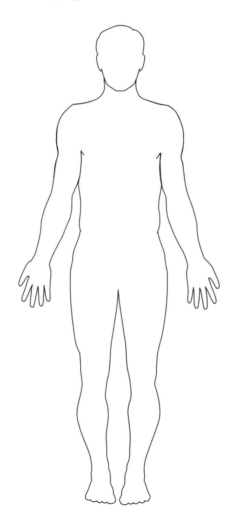

Collaborate and Share

In groups of 3 to 5 students, write 1 to 3 questions about the chapter on separate pieces of paper and crumple them into "snowballs." The instructor then mixes up the "snowballs" and throws them out to the groups, who then answer and discuss the questions within their group. If you get your own question back, return it to the instructor.

Explain and Learn

1. List everything you know about this chapter. As a group, pick 1 to 3 most important points and share with the class.

_____

_____

_____

_____

_____

_____

_____

_____

_____

2. Type on a separate sheet or handwrite below a sample Neuromuscular Review of Systems for a patient with some form of neuromuscular disease. Use as many of the terms from the word list in the chapter as appropriate. Explain why you included certain points. Remember to include both positives and negatives.

_____

_____

_____

_____

_____

_____

_____

Relax and Play

1. Form small groups and have each group select a different game show ("Who Wants to be a Millionaire," "Jeopardy," "Hollywood Squares," and so on) and create an "episode" using questions and answers related to this chapter. Use members from other groups as the contestants in your game show episode. The class can vote on the best presentation.

2. In small groups, draw a mind map on a piece of poster board, a large piece of butcher paper, or a brown paper grocery bag opened up and spread flat. Draw a circle in the center. In the main circle, place a word or phrase that represents the main point of the chapter. In the secondary or tertiary circles, put words or phrases that represent additional important points. With the members of the group, take turns tossing a coin onto the map. The person tossing the coin explains the term on which the coin landed (or nearest term). Continue until each term is discussed or until instructor calls "time."

Generalize and Apply

On a 3" x 5" card, write a statement of something you learned in this chapter and indicate how you think this information will help you in the study of this text or in the workplace. Give this card to your instructor as your "ticket out" of class today.

Compare and Contrast

1. Compare the neuromuscular system and the things that can go wrong with it to objects in your environment (plants, rocks, machines, furniture, buildings, etc.). How are they alike? How are they different?

_____

_____

_____

_____

2. Look up *syncope* and *seizure* in a medical dictionary. How does a syncopal episode differ from a seizure? How are they alike?

_____

_____

_____

_____

_____

Extrapolate and Project

Why must detailed information on symptoms suggestive of central nervous system disease sometimes be obtained from someone other than the patient? Who else might provide these details and under what circumstances?

_____

_____

_____

_____

_____

_____

_____

_____

_____

_____

13

Review of Systems: Psychiatric

This part of the Review of Systems is often omitted. The psychiatric history is even more intimate and sensitive, if possible, than the sexual history. A person with severe psychiatric impairment makes a most unreliable historian. For example, there is usually not much point in asking someone about a history of hallucinations or delusions, for these terms are used only by persons who are convinced of the unreality of the experiences. A person with even a mild mood or personality disorder frequently resists talking about it. Hence part or all of the psychiatric history may have to be obtained from the patient's family or friends or from medical records.

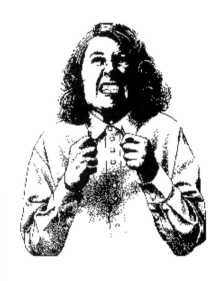

Psychiatric: No history of psychosis, anxiety or mood disorder, or hospitalization for nervous or mental disease.

Past history includes several psychiatric admissions for psychotic episodes consisting of auditory, visual, and tactile hallucinations and bizarre behavior.

Psychiatric history includes six admissions to the State Hospital because of inappropriate and threatening behavior, which frequently necessitated use of restraints.

anxiety   panic attacks   feeling of dread   agoraphobia   social phobia

jittery, jumpy, restless, tense, nervous   OCD (obsessive-compulsive disorder)

mood disorder   dysthymia   major, clinical depression   bipolar disorder

midlife crisis   *empty nest syndrome*

schizophrenia   delusions   hallucinations   dementia

conversion, hysteria, somatization

confusion, disorientation, delirium, *sundowning*

nightmares   sleepwalking, somnambulism   night terrors, pavor nocturnus

addiction, dependence, habituation, tolerance   substance abuse

anorexia nervosa, bulimia nervosa, eating disorder, pica

Alzheimer disease   toxic encephalopathy

Learning Objectives

After careful study of this chapter, you should be able to:

Distinguish between a psychiatric history and psychiatric exam.

Describe common psychiatric symptoms and diagnoses.

List common psychiatric treatment modalities.

Identify other areas of inquiry that would yield information about mental and emotional health.

At times it is hard to distinguish between psychiatric history-taking and psychiatric examination, since both make use of the same basic tool—interviewing the patient. When the patient's chief complaint is not psychiatric, inquiries about past or present mental illness or emotional disturbance are more clearly historical in intent. The interviewer asks about any prior diagnosis of mental, emotional, or nervous illness (anxiety, depression, social phobia, panic attacks, obsessive-compulsive disorder, bipolar disorder, schizophrenia, alcoholism, drug addiction),

For Quick Reference

addiction
agoraphobia
alcoholism
Alzheimer disease
anorexia nervosa
anxiety
auditory hallucination
bipolar disorder
bizarre behavior
bulimia nervosa
clinical depression
confusion
conversion
delirium
delusion
dementia
dependence
depression
disorientation
drug addiction
dysthymia
eating disorder
empty nest syndrome
habituation
hallucination
hysteria
inappropriate behavior
jittery
jumpy
major depression
mental disorder
midlife crisis
mood disorder
nervous disorder
neurosis
night terrors
nightmare
obsessive-compulsive disorder
panic attack
pavor nocturnus
pica
psychiatric impairment
psychosis
psychotic episode
restless
schizophrenia
sleepwalking
social phobia
somatization
somnambulism
substance abuse
sundowning
tactile hallucination
threatening behavior
tolerance
toxic encephalopathy
unreliable historian
visual hallucination

and treatments used, including counseling, group therapy, drug therapy, hospitalization, and electroshock. A general notion of the subject's mental and emotional health history can be obtained by inquiring about family and marital harmony, school performance, job stability and satisfaction, social contacts, sleep pattern, drug and alcohol use, and general sense of well-being, self-esteem, and purpose in life.

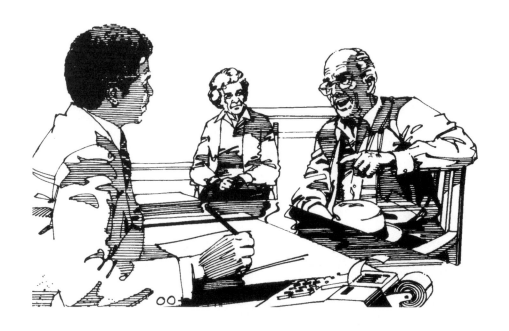

Exercises for Chapter 13

Review and Summarize

A. Fill in the Blank

1. A person with a severe psychiatric impairment is often a poor _____.

2. A medical doctor with special training in the diagnosis and treatment of mental illness is a(n)

_____.

3. The basic tool of the psychiatric history and physical exam is the _____.

B. Short Answer

1. What subjects might the physician discuss with the psychiatric patient in order to determine mental and emotional health?

_____

_____

_____

_____

_____

2. Why might the patient's medical record give a more reliable psychiatric history than the patient's own verbal report?

_____

_____

_____

_____

3. Write a short definition of the following terms. If you can, condense the definition into just a few words or a single synonym that you feel more comfortable with.

a. Hallucination _____

b. Anxiety_____

c. Phobia_____

d. Bipolar _____

e. Dysthymia_____

f. Delusion _____

g. Schizophrenia _____

h. Dementia_____

i. Somatization _____

j. Apathy_____

Pause and Reflect

Type on a separate sheet or handwrite below a Psychiatric Review of Systems for a character you know from a television show, movie, or book. Use as many of the terms from the chapter word list as are applicable.

_____

_____

_____

_____

_____

_____

_____

_____

_____

_____

_____

Relate and Remember

Create a flow chart or a diagram that illustrates how each part of the Psychiatric Review of Systems relates to the other parts.

Collaborate and Share

Label a blank sheet of paper with your name at the top and write a question requiring a short answer (less than a sentence) related to this chapter. Pass this paper to the student to your right, who will answer the question and then add a question of his or her own, as you answer the question on the paper received from the student on your left. Each sheet moves around the room until everyone has had a turn with every paper and you end up with the paper with your name at the top. Choose the best question(s) and answer(s) from your page to read aloud when called upon by your instructor.

Explain and Learn

Turn to the person next to you (or behind or in front of you), and share with each other one important piece of information you got from this chapter. Also share how you might use this information in your life or in your work. If you have a question that wasn't answered in the chapter, share that as well. If your partner doesn't have the answer, ask your instructor.

Relax and Play

1. On a 3" x 5" card, write a question pertaining to this chapter and give the card to your instructor. The instructor then tosses a koosh ball, small stuffed animal, net bath sponge, or some other soft object randomly to an individual student and reads a question from one of the cards. The student who caught the object must answer the question.

2. Role-play doctor and patient with another student and elicit a Psychiatric Review of Systems. Be sure to explore historical information and any current complaints, remembering that both positives and negatives are important. After doing this, switch roles and repeat the process, using different complaints/disease. Transcribe the information you elicited as a doctor.

Generalize and Apply

Make a mind map using the list of topics that appears in the last sentence of this chapter. For each of these topics, list as many psychiatric symptoms as you can think of that might be relevant to that topic. For example, under *sleep pattern*, restlessness and insomnia would be relevant symptoms.

Compare and Contrast

What is the difference between a *psychiatric exam* and *psychiatric history-taking*?

_____

_____

_____

_____

_____

_____

Extrapolate and Project

The author states that the terms *hallucinations* and *delusions* are used only by persons who are convinced of the unreality of the experiences. Explain in your own words what this means.

_____

_____

_____

_____

_____

_____

_____

_____

_____

_____

14

Review of Systems: Skin

The dermatologic history is usually omitted unless the patient has cutaneous complaints or a condition in which such complaints might be expected. The skin is subject to numerous injuries and local diseases and often reflects systemic disease as well.

> Skin: No history of itching, rash, nonhealing sores, or pigmented lesions.

The patient is questioned about prior diagnoses of severe or chronic cutaneous disease and any treatments used for them in the past or at present. Since patients often erroneously diagnose themselves as having psoriasis, fungal infection, or hives, the interviewer must be cautious in accepting such diagnoses. Lay persons are also prone to treat their own skin problems with a limitless variety of remedies, many of which can create further symptoms. Hence the physician inquires carefully about all such treatments.

> dermatitis, dermatosis   eczema
> atopic, contact, factitial, stasis dermatitis
> hives, urticaria   psoriasis
> athlete's foot, dermatophytosis, fungal infection, tinea, ringworm
> punch, skin biopsy   electrodesiccation
> **graft**: advancement, flap, full-thickness, partial-thickness

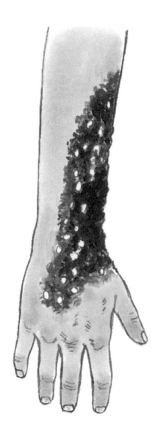

The commoner skin complaints are local or generalized eruptions or rashes, itching, dryness or scaling, pigment changes, and solid tumors of various kinds. Disorders of the hair (abnormal appearance of the hair, excessive hair, hair loss) and nails (deformity, discoloration) are also part of the dermatologic history. Lay persons are notoriously inept at describing their own skin lesions and rashes. If the problem is still present, the physician will usually not waste time in getting a garbled, secondhand description of something that is readily available for inspection.

> breaking out, eruption, exanthem, rash   itching, pruritus
> *galling*, intertrigo, irritation   dryness, roughness   flaking, scaling
> crust, eschar, scab   sore, ulcer
> black and blue marks, easy bruising, ecchymosis, extravasation

Learning Objectives

After careful study of this chapter, you should be able to:

Define the scope of the dermatologic Review of Systems.

List common symptoms of the skin, hair, and nails.

Describe the dermatologic history-taking process.

Identify terminology associated with the dermatologic Review of Systems.

Classify statements as belonging to the dermatologic Review of Systems.

For Quick Reference

athlete's foot
atopic dermatitis
beal
birthmark
blemish
boil
cicatrix
cicatrization
cold sore
comedo
contact dermatitis
cutaneous condition
dermatitis
dermatophytosis
dermatosis
ecchymosis
eczema
electrodesiccation
eruption
eschar
exanthem
extravasation
factitial dermatitis
festering
fever blister
fungal infection
hair loss
hirsutism
hives
hyperpigmented areas
intertrigo
mole
nevus
nonhealing sore
partial-thickness graft
pigmented lesion
pruritus
psoriasis
punch biopsy
pustule
ringworm
scab
scaling
scarring
skin biopsy
solid tumor
stasis dermatitis
suppuration
tinea
ulcer
urticaria
wart
weal, wheal
welp, whelp
welt
wen
zit

cold sore, fever blister   darkened, hyperpigmented areas

blemish, bump, comedo, pimple, pustule, spot, zit

beal, boil, festering, gathering, suppuration   *weal, welt*, wheal, *whelp, welp*

birthmark, mole, nevus, wart, *wen*   cicatrization, scarring

cold feet, burning feet

falling hair, thinning hair, excessive hair loss

excessive facial hair, hirsutism

cracked, discolored, splitting nails

But the physician will carefully question the patient about the duration of the problem; whether it comes and goes, remains unchanged, or is gradually getting better or worse; whether it is spreading from one area to others; whether the patient can suggest any reason for the problem; and whether anything seems to make the problem better or worse.

Exercises for Chapter 14

Review and Summarize

A. Multiple Choice

___ 1. All of the following are part of the dermatologic history EXCEPT
   a. Disorders of the hair.
   b. Disorders of the skin.
   c. Disorders of the lacrimal gland.
   d. Disorders of the nails.

___ 2. All of the following are used synonyms for "breaking out" EXCEPT
   a. Eruption.
   b. Eschar.
   c. Exanthem.
   d. Rash.

B. Fill in the Blank

1. Local disease of the skin often reflects the presence of _____ disease.

2. The dermatologic history is usually omitted unless the patient has _____ complaints.

C. Short Answer

1. List the five most common skin complaints.

   _____

   _____

   _____

2. What questions is the examiner likely to ask the patient complaining of a skin lesion?

   _____

   _____

   _____

   _____

3. Write a short definition of the following terms. If you can, condense the definition into just a few words or a single synonym that you feel more comfortable with.

a. Cutaneous _____

b. Psoriasis _____

c. Atopic _____

d. Eruption _____

e. Factitial _____

f. Electrodesiccation _____

g. Exanthem _____

h. Eschar _____

i. Hirsutism _____

j. Beal _____

k. Suppuration _____

l. Nevus _____

m. Cicatrix _____

Pause and Reflect

Have you or a member of your family ever had a skin condition which had cleared up significantly prior to a visit to the doctor? What terms did you use to describe your symptoms? With your knowledge of the questions a physician is likely to ask in a dermatologic Review of Systems, what information should you have been prepared to provide at your examination?

_____

_____

_____

_____

_____

Relate and Remember

Take a sheet of paper and draw lines to create four columns, labeled A through D. List five important things to remember about this chapter and put these in column A. In column B, next to each of the items to remember, write the name of an object that might help you to remember that fact. In column C, write the name of a place that might help you to remember that fact. In column D, write a description of a visual image with which you can associate the fact in column A.

Collaborate and Share

On a 3" x 5" card, write a question pertaining to this chapter. The instructor will divide the class into small groups and distribute some of the cards to each group. Within your group, discuss the questions you receive and agree on an answer for each question. Share your answers with the class.

Explain and Learn

Working in pairs, take turns pointing out and explaining the important points or main idea of each paragraph or section in this chapter.

Relax and Play

1. Fold a blank piece of paper in half three times so that when unfolded there are eight squares. Write one thing you learned in each square. Move around the room, asking other students to define or explain an item on your sheet. That student then signs the square. The student who gets all eight squares signed first wins.

2. Select 5 to 10 words or phrases from the word list in this chapter and create a word search puzzle. Rather than list the words you've chosen, however, provide definitions as clues. Copy the puzzles to share with the rest of the class. Students must first determine which word goes with the definition before finding it in the puzzle.

Generalize and Apply

On a sheet of paper, write a statement of something you learned in this chapter and how you think it will help you in your study of this book or in your work as a medical transcriptionist. Crumple up the sheet of paper to form a "snowball" and, along with other students in your class, toss it into the air and try to catch each other's snowballs. Read the statement from the snowball you caught to the rest of the class.

Compare and Contrast

Compare the skin and the things that can go wrong with it to objects in your environment (plants, machines, rocks, furniture, buildings, and so on). How are they alike? How are they different?

_____

_____

_____

_____

Extrapolate and Project

Draw a mind map with the name of a dermatologic diagnosis in the center circle, such as eczema, psoriasis, athlete's foot, tinea, urticaria, or intertrigo. In the next layer of circles, write the five questions listed in the last paragraph of this chapter. For each of these circles, write an answer based on the diagnosis you chose. Consult a medical dictionary or other textbooks if necessary. If you can't find an answer to a question, write a question mark in that circle. Show your completed map to your classmates and discuss your findings.

15

General Remarks on the Physical Examination

As with the history, the scope and character of the physical examination performed on a given patient in a given instance depend on circumstances. A Boy Scout camp physical may be rushed through in two or three minutes; thorough assessment of the nervous system alone in a patient suspected of having early multiple sclerosis can take more than an hour. Each physician performs a physical examination in the manner that personal experience has shown to be most efficient and convenient. Regardless of the sequence in which data are obtained, they are generally recorded in a format something like this:

General Appearance
Skin
Head and Face
Eyes
Ears
Nose, Throat, Mouth, Teeth
Neck
Thorax, Breasts, Axillae
Heart, Peripheral Vessels
Lungs
Abdomen, Groins, Anus, Rectum, Genitalia
Back and Extremities
Neurologic
Psychiatric

PE (physical examination, physical exam), physical

As mentioned in an earlier chapter, the term *physical examination* denotes, by convention, a group of diagnostic observations and maneuvers performed directly on the patient's body by the physician. Some of these maneuvers require the compliance or assistance of the patient and others do not. Only simple portable instruments are used. The following is a fairly comprehensive list of equipment used in the performance of a physical examination.

flashlight, head mirror, or
    other light source
magnifying glass
tape measure

diascope
clinical thermometer
watch with second hand
goniometer

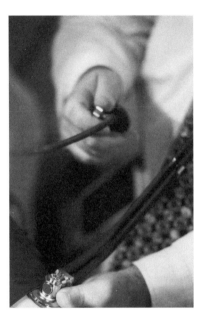

Learning Objectives

After careful study of this chapter, you should be able to:

Characterize the process by which a physical examination is performed and recorded.

Identify equipment employed in a physical examination.

Describe the four classical techniques of physical examination.

Explain the measurement of temperature, heart rate, and blood pressure.

Give examples of quantitative measurements used in a physical examination.

Describe the significant features of a mass and inflammation.

Identify terminology related to the physical examination.

For Quick Reference

A and P (auscultation and percussion)
accentuated
agenesis
angulation
anomalous
antigen-antibody reaction injury
apical pulse
aplasia, aplastic
asymmetry
atrophic thigh
atrophy, atrophic
atypical
augmented
auscultation
Babinski reflex
Babinski test
bacterial toxins injury
ballottable
ballottement
beefy red color
benign
blowing pansystolic murmur
BP (blood pressure)
burning injury
calor
cardiac rate
Celsius scale
centimeter
chemical irritants injury
congestion
contracted
crepitation
crepitus
crushing injury
cutting injury
cystic lesion
deficiency
deficit
deformed
deformity
development
deviation
diascope
diastolic pressure
dilated
diminished
discrete nodes
distorted
dolor
doughy mass
dysgenesis
dysmorphism
dysplasia, dysplastic
dystrophy, dystrophic
edema
electrical shock injury
enhanced
enlargement
erythema

ruler
tongue depressor
nasal speculum or rhinoscope
otoscope with various sizes
    of specula
ophthalmoscope
reflex hammer
sterile pin or needle
soft brush or cotton ball

skin-fold caliper
laryngeal mirror
tuning fork
stethoscope
sphygmomanometer
rubber gloves and lubricant
vaginal speculum
vision-testing chart

Virtually all diagnostic maneuvers employed in the physical examination are variations on four basic classical techniques: inspection (looking), palpation (feeling), auscultation (listening), and percussion (tapping). **Inspection** in medicine implies far more than just looking. A diagnostic inspection is objective, systematic, and thorough, with removal of clothing as needed, adequate lighting, and sometimes use of instruments to expose, illuminate, or magnify. The examiner correlates what is seen with other physical findings and with relevant details of the history. Inspection includes not only search and discovery but also recognition and interpretation.

Again, **palpation** goes far beyond mere prodding and pinching. The tactile sense of the trained diagnostician can detect and assess minute variations in the size, shape, and texture of organs and tissues, which are then related to visual impressions and other elements of the history and physical examination. Certain techniques and findings associated with palpation deserve special mention here. *Ballottement* (French, "shaking") is a technique of applying pressure intermittently to a body surface, somewhat as in bouncing a ball. By this means it is sometimes possible to detect deeply placed organs or masses that cannot otherwise be palpated. *Fluctuancy* refers to the tactile quality of confined fluid, as in a cyst, abscess, or swollen joint capsule. The palpating fingers can displace this fluid and perhaps even set up waves in it, as in compressing a balloon filled with water. *Fremitus* is a sensation of rubbing or vibration felt by the palpating fingers. It can be due to friction between two structures (such as a tendon and its sheath) or to transmission of sound (such as the patient's voice) through intervening tissues. *Crepitation* or *crepitus* is a grating or crackling sound produced by feeling or manipulating a part. Fremitus and crepitus sometimes occur together and the terms are not strictly distinguished in practice.

consistency, feel, texture	fluctuancy
crepitus, crepitation	pliable
ballottement, ballottable	fremitus

One common and very important physical finding hovers between symptom and sign: tenderness, which in medicine means a sensation of pain when pressure is applied to a part. Although elicited by the examiner's manipulations, tenderness is subjective, and its detection and assessment depend entirely on the patient's responses. Usually these responses are verbal, but even an infant or a semicomatose patient may betray tenderness by crying out or pulling away. Often the patient is already well aware that an area is abnormally sensitive and tries to prevent the examiner from touching it by moving away or grabbing the examiner's arm. Pain and tenderness often occur together, but in contrast to pain, which may be referred from a distant site, tenderness implies a local problem. Rebound tenderness, or pain on sudden release of the pressure of the examiner's hand on the abdomen, is characteristic of localized or generalized peritoneal irritation, implying some inflammatory process within the abdominal or pelvic cavity.

tenderness	*exquisitely* tender to palpation

tender to manipulation, palpation, pressure, touch
rebound, rebound tenderness
Any attempt at movement causes pain.
Abdominal palpation reveals no tenderness, rebound, spasm, or guarding.

Auscultation of internal organs is performed with a stethoscope, but the technique also includes listening to sounds produced by or in any part of the body. **Percussion**, first developed in the eighteenth century to assess the state of internal organs, particularly in the thorax, has become something of a lost art with the development of radiography, ultrasonography, computed tomography, magnetic resonance imaging, and various other types of noninvasive examination.

The lungs are clear to A and P (auscultation and percussion).

The rationale of physical examination rests on three basic assumptions: that there is such a thing as normality of bodily structure and function, corresponding to a state of health; that departures from this norm of structural and functional integrity consistently result from or correlate with specific abnormal states or diseases; and that systematic examination can detect these abnormalities and appraise them in such a way as to yield grounds for an accurate diagnosis.

What is normal? The term has two overlapping senses in medicine, which physicians seldom trouble to distinguish. First, normal means "usual, ordinary, average, common, unremarkable." In this sense, a condition or finding that is encountered in a majority of persons of a given sex and age would be considered normal. This type of normality can be established on a statistical basis, at least with respect to features or events that can be measured quantitatively, such as heart rate, ratio of height to weight, and age at onset of menstruation. Statistical analysis of measurements made in a large group of apparently healthy subjects shows that "normal" is never a single, absolute number but rather a range of numbers. This fact of biologic variation is acknowledged in such phrasing as "normal variant," "within normal limits," and "within the range of normal." From this perspective, *abnormal* means "anomalous, atypical, unusual, extraordinary," and sometimes "excessive" or "deficient."

Secondly, *normal* means "healthy, sound, intact, natural, unimpaired by disease or injury." It should be obvious that, in most medical contexts, *normal* (or

For Quick Reference

essentially negative
essentially normal
exaggerated
Fahrenheit degrees
feminization
fever
fibrous tissue (scar)
firm mass
fixation of mass to tissues
fixed mass
florid
fluctuancy
fluctuant mass
fluctuant nodes
fluid-filled mass
freely movable mass
freezing injury
fremitus
fullness
fulminant
function
fusiform mass
goniometer
guarding
hard mass
healing phase
heart murmurs
heightened
homogeneous mass
hyperemia
hyperplasia, hyperplastic
hyperpyrexia
hypertension
hypertrophy, hypertrophic
hypoplasia, hypoplastic
hypotension
ill-defined mass
impaired function
infantile
inflammatory process
inflammatory reaction
injection
inspection
intact
intensified
irregular mass
kilogram
Korotkoff sounds
labile hypertension
lack of mobility of mass
laesa functio (impaired function)
laryngeal mirror
lesion
lumpy mass
lymph nodes
malformation
malformed
maneuver

For Quick Reference

matted nodes
maturation
misshapen
mobility of mass
morbid
mushy mass
nondiagnostic
normal variant
normocephalic
normoglycemic
normotensive
ophthalmoscope
otoscope
overdeveloped
overgrown
palpation
pansystolic murmur
pathologic
pelvic examination
percentile rank
percussion
pitting edema
pliable
prostatic hypertrophy
pulse
pyrexia
radial pulse
rebound tenderness
rectal examination
redness
reflex hammer
resting pulse
right lower quadrant
Romberg test
roughly spherical mass
rubbery mass
rubedo
rubor
saccular mass
shotty nodes
skin-fold caliper
smooth mass
solid mass
solitary mass
spasm
spherical mass
sphygmomanometer
stable vital signs
stethoscope
stoic individual
stony hard mass
stony mass
structure
subcutaneous tissue
swelling
swollen calf
systolic pressure
tender to manipulation

---

appropriate, average, ordinary, unremarkable, usual

no significant abnormalities   within normal limits, range   normal variant

atypical, anomalous

---

abnormal) applies equally in both senses. Moreover, physicians often use the term *negative* interchangeably with *normal*. *Negative* implies the lack or absence of something. Since the diagnostician is searching for abnormalities, the term *negative* may seem appropriate when a particular line of inquiry fails to turn up any: "The family history is negative for hypertension." "The left breast is entirely negative," "Rectal examination is negative." The expression, "The Romberg is negative," is shorthand for "The Romberg test yields a negative (normal, expected) result." "The Babinski is negative" means, "The Babinski reflex (which would be abnormal if present) is absent." (Conversely, *positive* often implies *abnormal*: "positive Romberg," "positive findings in the fundus.") The ubiquitous phrases *essentially normal* and *essentially negative* mean "sound, unimpaired, normal with allowance for expected and insignificant variations."

---

essentially negative, normal   nondiagnostic

intact, unimpaired

no evidence of disease or injury   no *pathology* found

abnormal, diseased, morbid, pathologic

Abdominal exam is benign.   normocephalic, normoglycemic, normotensive

Extraocular muscles are grossly intact.

Examination is confined (limited, restricted) to the left knee.

examination demonstrates, discloses, indicates, reveals, shows

---

A physical examination is a set of standard procedures intended to detect and appraise any significant departures from normal. The living body and its parts can be normal or abnormal in two basic ways: in structure and in function. *Structure* here includes all static features that are subject to examination, assessment, or measurement by an observer, such as height, weight, and girth; shape, size, and symmetry of parts or organs; color, texture, and integrity of surfaces. *Function* includes any physiologic or pathologic action or capacity for action of a bodily tissue, organ, region, or system that can be tested or evaluated by an observer, such as the pupillary reflex to light, hearing acuity, cardiac rate, muscle strength,

---

mild, minimal, slight   apparent, detectable, evident, obvious

considerable, moderate, substantial

extreme, marked, massive, severe   florid, fulminant, obvious

finding, observation   condition, quality, state

accentuated, augmented, dilated, enhanced, enlarged, exaggerated, heightened, increased, intensified

contracted, diminished, limited, lowered, reduced

and the ability to stand upright without swaying or falling. Although a disturbance of function generally arises from structural alteration, it does not follow that every departure from the expected structure results in functional impairment.

Several general concepts must be defined or explained in preparation for the discussion of specific techniques of physical examination to be presented in later chapters. First, an examiner always considers the state of *development* of a subject. Development can be expressed in purely numerical terms, as when a child's height and weight are given a percentile rank on the basis of measurements of thousands of children of the same chronologic age, or when arm span is expressed as a fraction of height. Development may also refer to the configuration of a part or of the body as a whole. Lack of symmetry or other obvious deviation from the expected shape of the head, the trunk, or some other part often, but not always, indicates a flaw in development, possibly genetically determined or due to birth injury. Development may also refer to the attainment of a certain stage of maturation, such as the appearance of secondary sexual characteristics at puberty.

For Quick Reference

tender to palpation
tender to pressure
tender to touch
tongue depressor
tumescence
tumor
tuning fork
unable to cooperate
uncooperative
underdeveloped
unimpaired
vaginal speculum
viral invasion
virilization
vision-testing chart
within normal limits
woody mass

> development   maturation
> hypoplastic, infantile, underdeveloped
> absent, missing   agenesis
> hyperplastic, hypertrophic, overdeveloped, overgrown
> aplasia, dysplasia, hyperplasia, hypoplasia
> atrophy, dystrophy, hypertrophy
> deformity, dysgenesis, dysmorphism, malformation   asymmetry
> deficiency, deficit   angulation, deviation
> anomalous, deformed, distorted, malformed, misshapen
> virilization, feminization

A visible or palpable abnormality that represents more than a mere malformation or quantitative deviation from expected structure may be called a lesion (Latin *laesio* "injury"). Physicians apply this generic term not only to the results of injury but also to abnormal masses and inflammatory or degenerative processes, particularly when these are readily visible on skin or mucous membranes. They may even use it in an abstract sense, as in "the biochemical lesion of diabetes mellitus."

> Examination of the entire skin surface reveals no lesions.
> a cystic lesion measuring 2 x 3 cm

An abnormal mass can occur in any part of the body, and can be a benign or malignant growth, a malformed or enlarged organ, a product of inflammation, or a foreign body, to name the most likely possibilities. Lymph nodes, many of which lie in the fat layer under the skin, particularly in the neck, axillae, and groins, quite commonly enlarge and become palpable in response to various local and systemic processes, most often infectious or malignant. The discovery of a mass can be particularly ominous and can place the physician in an awkward dilemma. Absolute certainty as to the nature of a mass can seldom be arrived at without removal of part

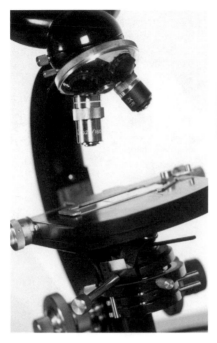

or all of it for microscopic examination; but such removal can lead to serious functional impairment or mutilation. Hence every mass demands the most diligent evaluation.

A smooth, roughly spherical mass is palpable in the right lower quadrant.
(lymph) nodes: discrete, fluctuant, matted, shotty

The features of a mass that require consideration, besides its exact anatomic location and relationships, are its size, shape, texture, mobility, and the presence or absence of pulsations or tenderness. Many possible variations, all highly meaningful, come under the heading of texture: a mass can be smooth and homogeneous, or lumpy and irregular; stony hard (suggesting calcification or malignancy), firm, rubbery, doughy, or mushy; solid or fluctuant (containing fluid that shifts on manipulation of the mass). A fluid-filled mass is usually referred to as a cyst. Mobility refers to the freedom with which a mass can be shifted about by manipulation; lack of mobility implies continuity with surrounding tissues, or fixation to them (another clue to malignancy).

mass: doughy, firm, fixed, fluctuant, fusiform, hard, (freely) movable, mushy, rubbery, saccular, smooth, solitary, stony, woody
a 2. 5 cm ill-defined but roughly spherical mass just below the right scapular angle, moving with the subcutaneous tissue and apparently fixed in the skin

The term *inflammation* refers to one of the cardinal concepts of pathology. **Inflammation** is a stereotyped pattern of biochemical, hematological, and mechanical events that occur in living tissue in response to injury of any kind, whether due to cutting, crushing, burning, freezing, electrical shock, chemical irritants, bacterial toxins, viral invasion, or antigen-antibody reactions. Although the precise nature of an inflammatory reaction depends on the type and extent of the cause and the tissue involved, the basic features are the same—local production or release of various complex chemical substances, dilatation of capillaries, and migration of fluid and cells from the blood to the tissues. These chemical and histologic events account for the gross manifestations of inflammation, described by the first-century medical writer Celsus in terms that remain valid today: *rubor* (redness), *tumor* (swelling), *calor* (heat), and *dolor* (pain). Medieval physicians added

congestion, erythema, hyperemia, injection, redness, rubedo, rubor
angry, beefy red color
edema, enlargement, fullness, swelling, tumescence, tumor
firm, hard, indurated, tough   friable
calor, fever, heat, warmth
ache, pain, soreness, tenderness
cicatrix, fibrosis, scar, scarring, scar tissue   keloid
granulation (tissue)   granuloma

laesa functio (impaired function). The Latin terms are still occasionally used today. An inflammatory process usually passes in time into a healing phase, during which significant damage to tissue may be repaired with a patch of fibrous tissue (scar).

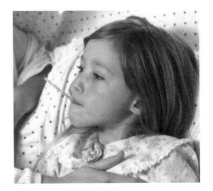

In assessing function, the physician may instruct the examinee to perform a certain activity, such as standing erect with eyes closed, or may carry out a test that requires no voluntary cooperation, such as stroking the sole of the examinee's foot and noting the response. Most of these maneuvers have eponymic names, like the Romberg and Babinski tests just described.

The Romberg is negative
Babinskis are *downgoing*.

Quantitative measurements play an essential role in physical diagnosis. The basic physical examination includes measurements of height, weight, temperature, pulse (heart rate), respiratory rate, and blood pressure, which are usually included at the beginning of the physical examination report. To an increasing extent, height and weight are recorded in metric units (centimeters and kilograms) in this country. **Temperature** is still generally recorded in Fahrenheit degrees, though the Celsius scale is used at a few medical centers. Temperature is taken orally except when the patient's age or condition makes the rectal route preferable.

Height 5'8½" (174 cm)	Temperature 99.2°F (37.2°C) orally
Weight 142# (142 lb.) (64.5 kg)	Rectal temperature 102.6°
fever, hyperpyrexia, pyrexia	(elevated) temperature

Heart rate is recorded in beats per minute. Unless the cardiac rhythm is irregular the examiner usually counts beats for only 15 seconds and multiplies by four. The heart rate may be counted as pulsations in a peripheral artery, most often the radial artery at the wrist (radial pulse) or as beats heard with a stethoscope placed on the chest near the cardiac apex (apical pulse). The respiratory rate, recorded as respirations per minute, is also usually determined by 15 seconds' actual observation. The examiner usually counts respirations while ostensibly doing something else, e.g., still feeling the pulse at the wrist. This is because the awareness that one's breathing is being observed makes it almost impossible to breathe at a natural rate and depth.

Vital signs are stable.	
cardiac rate, heart rate, pulse	
resting pulse	76 and regular
apical pulse 84	81 with frequent PVC's

Blood pressure is determined in the brachial artery above the elbow with the help of a stethoscope and a sphygmomanometer. The latter consists of an inflatable cuff with a pressure gauge. The cuff is wrapped around the subject's arm and

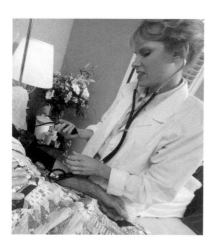

inflated until no pulsations are transmitted from the heart to the artery below the cuff. While listening to this artery with a stethoscope, the examiner then slowly deflates the cuff, noting the pressure at which pulsations can just be heard, and the somewhat lower pressure at which they cease to be audible. The higher of these readings is taken as the maximum pressure attained by the blood in response to a contraction of the heart (systolic pressure); the lower, the pressure to which the blood drops between contractions (diastolic pressure). By convention, these figures are reported as a fraction, with the higher number on top, e.g., 120/80, pronounced "one twenty over eighty." In certain circumstances blood pressure may be taken with the cuff applied to the thigh.

BP (blood pressure)	175/110
Korotkoff sounds	hypertension; hypotension
Blood pressure is unobtainable.	labile hypertension

Other quantitative measurements may be appropriate in the course of an examination—for example, determination of heart rate immediately after exercise, comparison of the diameter of a swollen calf or an atrophic thigh with that of the normal one, or measurement of a scar, a zone of redness, or a mass. Certain phenomena, such as heart murmurs, are graded numerically. A common way for an examiner to record the extent or degree of a finding is to grade it on an arbitrary scale of 1+ to 4+. Comparison to the size of a familiar object ("about the size of a walnut"), though homely and imprecise, is also widely used.

a grade 2 blowing pansystolic murmur
2+ pitting edema of both ankles
4+ prostatic hypertrophy
a patch of erythema about the size of a dime

In performing a physical examination, the physician strives for rigor and thoroughness while seeking to keep the patient relaxed and comfortable. Often these goals are incompatible. Some parts of the examination inevitably generate fear, embarrassment, or pain, at least for some subjects. The attendance of a nurse or aide who can help the patient to remove clothing or assume certain positions while providing emotional support is sometimes essential. A gown or sheet or both can be used to cover parts of the body not presently being examined. A female attendant is customarily present when a male physician examines a woman patient.

In recording findings on physical examination, the physician makes note of any factors that have limited the thoroughness or reliability of the examination,

uncooperative, unable to cooperate
It is somewhat difficult to gauge the severity of this episode because she is a quite stoic individual and at all times tends to minimize her symptoms.
Pelvic and rectal examinations are deferred.

such as the patient's inability to cooperate because of lethargy, pain, or fear. If any standard part of the examination procedure is abridged, modified, or omitted, that fact is recorded, so that anyone reading the report of the examination will not falsely assume that it was done.

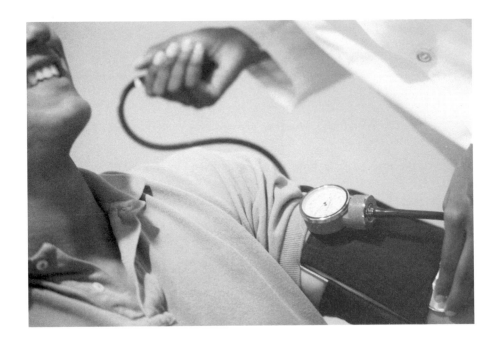

Exercises for Chapter 15

Review and Summarize

Multiple Choice

___ 1. The body's response to injury with redness, swelling, and pain is termed
      a. Infection.
      b. Infarction.
      c. Inflammation.
      d. Induration.

___ 2. Which of the following is NOT one of the four basic techniques of the physical examination?
      a. Inspection.
      b. Percussion.
      c. Palpation.
      d. Perfusion.
      e. Auscultation.

___ 3. Crepitus is
      a. A grating or crackling sound.
      b. The sensation of rubbing or vibration.
      c. Deterioration.
      d. Friction.

___ 4. Auscultation is performed with
      a. The examiner's hands.
      b. A magnifying glass.
      c. A stethoscope.
      d. A reflex hammer.
      e. A light source.

Fill in the Blank

1. _____ is a French term that means "shaking."

2. The tactile quality of a confined fluid is known as _____.

3. Pain on sudden release of the examiner's hand on the abdomen is called _____ tenderness.

4. A fluid-filled mass is usually referred to as a(n) _____.

5. Blood pressure is usually taken at the _____ artery.

6. The lower number of a blood pressure reading is the _____ pressure.

Short Answer

1. Write a short definition of the following terms. If you can, condense the definition into just a few words or a single synonym that you feel more comfortable with.

   a. Caliper _____

   b. Diascope _____

   c. Sphygmomanometer _____

   d. Ophthalmoscope _____

   e. Rationale _____

   f. Ominous _____

   g. Static _____

   h. Lesion _____

   i. Quantitative _____

   j. Fremitus _____

   k. Anomalous _____

   l. Virilization _____

   m. Fusiform _____

   n. Tumescence _____

2. A sample format is introduced at the beginning of this chapter. By what method are the categories arranged?

   _____

   _____

   _____

   _____

   _____

   _____

Pause and Reflect

Using different colored highlighters or crayons, underline or highlight important points or main ideas of the chapter. Circle key words. Use symbols (such as stars, asterisks, exclamation points, question marks) meaningful to you to mark key words and phrases. Summarize in your own words the information you thought most important from the chapter. If you have any questions, write those out to share with classmates or to ask your instructor.

_____

_____

_____

_____

_____

Relate and Remember

1. Think of a metaphor that completes this statement: A thorough and reliable physical examination is like a _____. Use a visual or a verbal metaphor. You may fill in the blank with the name of an object or draw (or cut out of a magazine) a picture representing one or more important points. Explain your choice.

_____

_____

_____

_____

_____

_____

_____

_____

_____

_____

2. Create a visual representation of the entire physical examination report. You may use a drawing, flow chart, graph, diagram, or metaphorical illustration. Explain, if necessary, how the visual representation relates to the physical exam.

Collaborate and Share

After you have read the chapter, form groups of 3 to 5. Divide the chapter so that each group has a portion. Re-read your section. As a group, write questions based on your section. They may be multiple choice, short answer, or fill in the blank. The number of questions will depend on how large a section of the chapter your group is covering. Pass your questions to the next group, working clockwise around the room, until every group has had the opportunity to answer all the questions.

Explain and Learn

In groups of 3 to 5 students, with each group assigned a different section of the chapter, discuss and agree on the important points or main ideas. Put them into your own words. Select one person to present your summary to the class.

Relax and Play

1. After reviewing the chapter as a class or in small groups, the instructor will announce "Go," and individual class members will "pop up" and call out one important fact learned, already known, or remembered about a topic or section in this chapter.

2. Individually or in groups, pantomime a diagnostic maneuver or procedure, such as ballottement, assessing a mass, taking blood pressure, and so on. Explain what you are doing, what you are looking for, and what you are finding as you go along.

Generalize and Apply

Draw a mind map with "physical examination" in the center circle. Draw 14 secondary circles and fill in the headings from the list that appears at the beginning of this chapter. For each of these headings draw 3 to 5 additional circles and write the name of an examination instrument or technique that a physician might employ. For example, for the abdomen, you might include stethoscope, palpation, ballottement, and so on.

Compare and Contrast

Fremitus and *crepitus* are similar sounding terms with similar meanings. Discuss how you would differentiate between these terms if encountered in dictation.

_____

_____

_____

_____

_____

Extrapolate and Project

The author states that keeping a patient relaxed and comfortable while performing a rigorous and thorough physical examination are often incompatible goals. If a patient experiences fear, embarrassment, or pain during a physical examination, what specific limitations does this impose on the examining physician? What impact, if any, would there be on the findings obtained on examination?

_____

_____

_____

_____

_____

_____

_____

_____

_____

_____

16

General Appearance

The physical examination report usually begins with a description of the patient's general appearance. To the experienced examiner, the first glance at a patient conveys volumes of information. Before the history is finished, many features of the patient's overall appearance will have been observed, and definite opinions about the general state of mental and physical health will have been formed. In carrying out the physical examination, the diagnostician has opportunities to make further observations and to confirm or correct those impressions before committing them to writing.

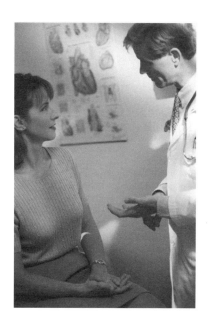

> Physical examination reveals a normally developed and nourished white male appearing the stated age of 54, who is alert, cheerful, cooperative, and in no acute distress.
>
> The patient is awake, alert, nontoxic-appearing, eupneic, and in no distress.

The general features noted by the diagnostician in performing a physical examination include body build (muscular development, proportions, skeletal deformities), nutritional status, apparent age and general state of health, skin color (pallor, cyanosis, jaundice), alertness and responsiveness, mood, posture, gait, mobility, grooming and personal hygiene, quality and clarity of voice and speech, evidence of distress (shortness of breath, signs of pain or anxiety), abnormal odors of breath or body, and any other readily observable abnormalities (facial scars, absence of a limb).

build, habitus, physique   torso, trunk
development, proportions   asthenic, pyknic
dysmorphism, deformity   ectomorphic, endomorphic, mesomorphic
cretinism, dwarfism, gargoylism, gigantism, mongolism
achondroplasia   acromegaly   arachnodactyly, Marfan syndrome
cushingoid, eunuchoid, marfanoid   *buffalo hump*
virilization, feminization
obese, overnourished, overweight
adiposity, female-pattern, male-pattern, truncal obesity
thin, slender, slim, skinny, malnourished, undernourished
cachectic, emaciated, marantic, wasted
cachexia, emaciation, marasmus, wasting

Learning Objectives

After careful study of this chapter, you should be able to:

Explain the importance of the general appearance to the diagnostic process.

Classify general and specific features documented in the general appearance.

Identify terminology descriptive of a patient's general appearance.

Give examples of contributing clues and impressions that may be unrecorded.

For Quick Reference

action tremor
air hunger
alcoholic breath
ammoniacal odor
antalgic gait
apneustic breathing
apraxic gait
atactic breathing
babbling speech
Biot breathing
blood-streaked sputum
blue bloater
brassy cough
bubbling cough
carphologia
carpopedal spasm
Cheyne-Stokes breathing
chrysoderma
circumoral pallor
cloudy sensorium
croupy cough
cyanosis, cyanotic
decerebrate rigidity
decorticate rigidity
decreased I:E ratio
diaphoresis, diaphoretic
dysarthric speech
dyspnea, dyspneic
expiratory phase
festinating gait
fetal position
fetid odor
flat(tened) affect
foul odor
frothy sputum
fruity breath
garbled speech
gelatinous sputum
glue-footed gait
habit spasm
hacking cough
halitosis
halting speech
harsh cough
hemiballismus
hemiplegic gait
hollow cough
hydrops
hyperpnea
hyperventilation
hysterical gait
icterus, icteric
inspiratory phase
intention tremor
jerky speech
ketotic breath
Kussmaul breathing
lisping speech

anasarca, hydrops, dropsy

fit, hale, healthy, hearty, robust, sound   frail, feeble

acutely ill, chronically ill   *toxic, shocky*

in extremis, moribund

beet red, beefy red, florid, flushed, plethoric   malar flush

pink puffer   circumoral pallor

ashen, cadaverous, pale, pallid, sallow, waxy, pallor, paleness

cyanotic, leaden, livid

cyanosis: central, generalized, peripheral

blue bloater   pickwickian

chrysoderma, icterus, jaundice

diaphoretic, perspiring, sweating   anhidrotic

drooling   retarded

alert, normally oriented, well-oriented   apathetic

comatose, confused, dazed   flat(tened) affect

cloudy sensorium, disoriented, obtunded, stuporous, unresponsive

apprehensive, anxious, cranky, depressed, euphoric, hostile, irritable, resentful, tearful, tense, uncooperative

posture, stance, station   fetal position

decorticate, decerebrate rigidity   opisthotonos

kyphotic   slumped   stiff neck   poker, rigid spine

akinetic, hypoactive   lies tense and still with knees drawn up

hyperkinetic, hyperactive, hypermobile   moves all extremities well

fidgety   writhing   *carphologia*

carpopedal spasm   tetany   in restraints

myoclonus   myokymia

hemiballismus   tic, twitch, habit spasm

chorea   athetosis

fasciculation, fibrillation   asterixis, *liver flap*

tremor: action, intention, pill-rolling, postural, resting, static, ambulant, ambulatory

limping, reeling, staggering, weaving

gait: antalgic, apraxic, festinating, *glue-footed*, hemiplegic, hysterical, propulsion, scissors, shuffling, spastic, steppage, Trendelenburg, waddling, wide-based

grooming, personal hygiene

aphasia, dysarthria   mute   dysphonia, hoarseness

voice: hoarse, hollow, *hot-potato*, nasal, weak   stammer, stutter

speech: babbling, dysarthric, indistinct, garbled, halting, jerky, lisping, monotonous, muttered, pressured, rapid, scanning, slurred, stuttering

air hunger, breathlessness, dyspnea, respiratory distress, respiratory embarrassment, shortness of breath

hyperpnea, tachypnea

breath: alcoholic, fruity, ketotic, mousy, musty   halitosis

odor: ammoniacal, fetid, foul, putrid, septic   odor of urine, sweat

Some of these features are evident merely on inspection, some require more elaborate techniques, perhaps involving the collaboration of the patient, and some depend on inference. Although the physician's appraisal of a patient's general condition is often reduced to a formula in the physical examination report, it is safe to say that in most cases a number of unrecorded and perhaps not consciously noticed impressions and clues contribute to the overall diagnostic conclusions.

A comparison between the apparent and actual ages provides a broad general notion of the patient's lifestyle, state of nutrition, and general medical condition. Obesity can be quantified to some extent by measurement of skin folds at selected standard sites with a caliper or by the application of a formula relating weight to height. Facial expression, speech, and manner offer clues to the patient's mental state as well as to the integrity of the central nervous system. Some of the physician's observations and conclusions about alertness, orientation, and emotional equilibrium will go into the record of the psychiatric (mental status) examination, if one is made. Some of them may even be noted at the beginning of the history if the examiner believes that they have affected the completeness or accuracy of the patient's responses.

> Skin fold measured over the midtriceps is 3.5 cm.

The patient's body posture, stance, mobility, and gait are of particular interest during the orthopedic and neurologic examinations, but gross abnormalities such as hemiparesis, spinal rigidity, tremors, or a shuffling or staggering gait will be noted as part of the general appearance. Speech can be rendered abnormal by a disorder of the mouth, tongue, pharynx, or larynx that alters the quality of the voice or interferes with the articulation of words, or by brain or nerve disease that impairs the normal function of the vocal cords and speech apparatus. A stroke can completely abolish the faculty of speech (aphasia).

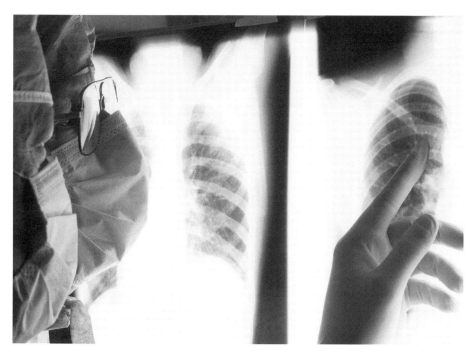

For Quick Reference

liver flap
loose cough
malar flush
metallic cough
monotonous speech
mousy breath
musty breath
muttered speech
nonproductive cough
nontoxic-appearing
normally developed and nourished white male
normally oriented
opisthotonous
peripheral cyanosis
pickwickian syndrome
pill-rolling tremor
pink puffer
poker spine
postural tremor
pressured speech
productive cough
propulsion gait
purulent sputum
putrid odor
putrid sputum
rapid speech
rasping cough
rattling cough
respiratory embarrassment
respiratory stertor
respiratory stridor
resting tremor
rigid spine
ropy sputum
rusty sputum
scanning speech
scissors gait
septic odor
shallow breathing
shuffling gait
singultus
slurred speech
spastic gait
staggering gait
static tremor
steppage gait
stertorous breathing
stridulous breathing
stuttering speech
tachypnea, tachypneic
Trendelenburg gait
viscid sputum
viscous sputum
waddling gait
watery sputum
wide-based gait
wracking cough

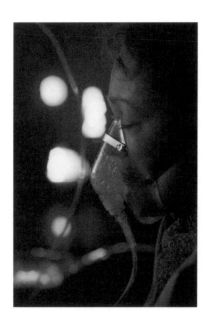

Respiratory distress and cough are also sufficiently conspicuous features to be noted here. The examiner observes whether dyspnea is accompanied by audible wheezing, cough, or production of froth or sputum, and whether it is less severe in the upright position. The rhythm of breathing is also noted, as well as the quality of cough. Observations as to the patient's tolerance for pain ("pain threshold") may be appropriately included here.

breathing, respiration   apnea

eupneic   tachypneic   bradypneic   orthopneic

hyperpnea, hyperventilation

breathing: apneustic, atactic, Biot, Cheyne-Stokes, Kussmaul, shallow, sighing, stertorous, stridulous

respiratory stertor, stridor   wheezing   choking, gasping   decreased *I:E ratio*

prolonged inspiratory, expiratory phase   hiccups, singultus

cough: brassy, bubbling, croupy, hacking, harsh, hollow, loose, metallic, nonproductive, productive, rasping, rattling, wracking

sputum: blood-streaked, frothy, gelatinous, green, purulent, putrid, ropy, rusty, viscid, viscous, watery yellow

high, low (pain) threshold

Exercises for Chapter 16

Review and Summarize

A. Multiple Choice

___ 1. A person with aphasia is
   a. Unable to urinate.
   b. Unable to swallow.
   c. Unable to speak.
   d. Unable to breathe.

___ 2. What can the physician ascertain about a patient even before completion of the history-taking?
   a. General state of mental health.
   b. General state of physical health.
   c. Both "a" and "b."
   d. Nothing.

B. Fill in the Blank

1. The patient's state of alertness, orientation, and emotional equilibrium goes into the record of the

   _____examination, if one is made.

2. Facial expression, speech, and manner offer clues to the patient's _____.

C. Short Answer

1. List general features noted by the physician when performing a physical examination.

   _____

   _____

   _____

   _____

   _____

   _____

2. Write a short definition of the following terms. If you can, condense the definition into just a few words or a single synonym that you feel more comfortable with.

a. Habitus _____

b. Asthenic _____

c. Pyknic _____

d. Cushingoid _____

e. Marantic _____

f. Cachexia _____

g. Obtunded _____

h. Adiposity _____

i. Stridor _____

j. Purulent _____

k. Anasarca _____

l. Diaphoretic _____

m. Festinating gait _____

Pause and Reflect

Read this chapter aloud, by yourself or taking turns with other students. If you don't know the meaning or pronunciation of a word, you should look it up. As you read, pause and reflect on key points at the end of each section. Make notes in the margins of your book, mark with dots or stars, and draw lines from key ideas to subordinate points. Summarize your reading in outline form.

_____

_____

_____

_____

_____

_____

Relate and Remember

Using this outline of the human body, list 3 to 5 terms for each area that the physician might use to describe the general appearance.

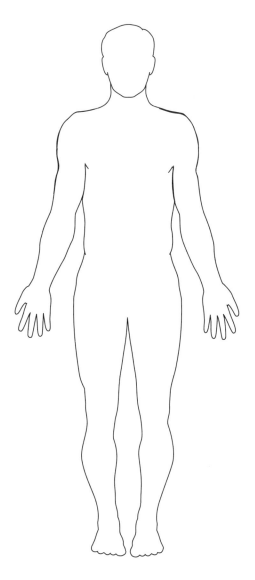

Collaborate and Share

In groups of 3 to 5 students, write 1 to 3 questions about the chapter on separate pieces of paper and crumple them into "snowballs." The instructor then mixes up the "snowballs" and throws them out to the groups, who then answer and discuss the questions within their group. If you get your own question back, return it to the instructor.

Explain and Learn

Type on a separate sheet or handwrite below a sample general appearance examination for a patient with a disease whose symptoms are familiar to you. Use as many of the terms from the word list in the chapter as appropriate. Explain why you included certain points. Remember to include both positives and negatives.

_____

_____

_____

_____

_____

_____

_____

_____

_____

_____

_____

_____

Relax and Play

1. Form small groups and have each group select a different game show ("Who Wants to be a Millionaire," "Jeopardy," "Hollywood Squares," and so on) and create an "episode" using questions and answers related to this chapter. Use members from other groups as the contestants in your game show episode. The class can vote on the best presentation.

2. Select 10 to 20 words or phrases from the word list in this chapter. Write a poem or song that incorporates these terms in such a way as to reveal both their meaning and use. If writing a song, you can use a familiar tune or rap style.

Generalize and Apply

Draw a mind map with "General Appearance" in the center circle. Using the list of general features that appears in the second paragraph of this chapter, fill in the secondary circles. In the next ring of circles, list 3 to 5 adjectives for each general feature, taken from the word list accompanying this chapter. Begin a fourth ring of circles, supplying one additional adjective not appearing in this chapter for every adjective in the third ring. If you have trouble thinking of additional adjectives, look up the definitions for terms in the word list to find antonyms and synonyms.

Compare and Contrast

A physician will compare the patient's apparent and actual ages to gain a broad general notion of the patient's lifestyle, state of nutrition, and general medical condition. For each of these three categories, discuss the conclusions the physician might make if the patient appears much older than the stated age. How would these conclusions differ if the patient's appearance matched his or her age? How would they differ if the patient appeared much younger than the stated age?

_____

_____

_____

_____

_____

_____

Extrapolate and Project

The author notes that in most cases a number of unrecorded and perhaps not consciously noticed impressions and clues contribute to the overall diagnostic conclusions. Discuss what type of information might be unrecorded but contribute to the diagnosis. Can you think of impressions and clues that might not be consciously noticed? Give examples.

_____

_____

_____

_____

_____

_____

_____

_____

_____

_____

_____

17

Examination of the Skin

Dermatologists like to say that the skin is the largest and most conspicuous organ of the body. No one would dispute the latter half of that assertion. Not only is the whole of the skin accessible for examination, but the skin is interposed between the examiner and most of the bodily structures that need to be assessed. With a few exceptions, inspecting the body means looking at skin. Hence the diagnostician is almost constantly observing the skin for evidence of injury or disease, no matter what region is being examined.

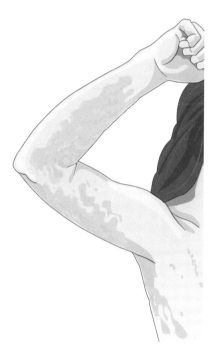

> The skin is clear.
> cutis, dermis, skin   epidermis   corium
> glabrous, hairy skin   keratin   stratum corneum
> mucocutaneous   subcutaneous tissue

Cutaneous diagnosis depends on a consideration of many factors: the type, number, grouping, and location of lesions; combinations of features occurring together; signs of evolutionary change, secondary infection, or the effects of treatment; and the presence of associated symptoms such as fever, headache, or pain in the joints or abdomen. While many skin problems (acne, warts, poison ivy, ringworm) arise in the skin and stay there, many others (hives, the eruptions of chickenpox and lupus erythematosus) are signs of systemic disease.

> dermatitis, dermatosis   eczema
> erythema multiforme   erythema nodosum
> **dermatitis**: atopic, contact, factitial, stasis   centrifugal, centripetal
> oozing, seeping, weeping   linear   annular, circinate
> plaque   blotchy, patchy, scattered, streaky   Christmas-tree pattern
> *bull's eye*, iris, *target* lesions   guttate   notched, scalloped, serpiginous
> hyperkeratosis, keratosis, porokeratosis   keratin plugs
> herpetiform, scarlatiniform, morbilliform   satellite lesions
> eruption, exanthem, rash
> sharply marginated violaceous plaques with imbricated, closely adherent, silvery scales
> intertrigo, chafing, galling   granulation tissue, granuloma, proud flesh
> dimple, fistula, sinus tract   eczematization
> 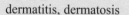 draining sinus   foreign body

Learning Objectives

After careful study of this chapter, you should be able to:

Name the factors affecting cutaneous diagnosis.

Define 20 basic skin lesions.

Describe distribution patterns of lesions.

Identify terminology related to the skin, hair, and nails.

Classify H&P statements as belonging to the skin exam.

For Quick Reference

abrasion
abscess
acne
ala nasi
albinism
alopecia
angioedema
angioneurotic edema
anhidrosis
atopic dermatitis
atrophy
Beau lines
bedsore
bleb (bulla)
blunt trauma
brawny edema
bronzing
bull's eye lesion
bursting-type laceration
café au lait spot
callus, callosity
calvities
canities
capillary dilatation
capillary fragility
carbuncle
caseous drainage
castlike desquamation
cavernous hemangioma
cellulitis
chancre
cheesy drainage
cherry angioma
chilblain
chloasma
Christmas-tree pattern
chrysoderma
cicatrix
closed wound
clustered distribution of lesions
comedo
concave drumstick nails
condyloma acuminatum
confluent distribution of lesions
contact dermatitis
contact ulcer
contusion
corium
crater
curdy drainage
cutaneous diagnosis
cutis
cyanosis (blueness)
cyst
debris
decubitus ulcer
depigmentation
dermal appendages

gangrene	necrosis
ringworm, tinea	impetigo, impetiginization
Nikolsky sign	Koebner phenomenon
minute vesicles in streaks and clusters on an erythematous base	
Osler nodes	Janeway spots
tophus	lipoma

In assessing the skin, the physician ensures adequate exposure of the surface by removing clothing, dressings, bandages, and ointments and by using bright natural or artificial light and, as needed, a magnifying lens. Examination of the skin is not carried out by inspection alone. The examiner palpates any area of skin that appears abnormal and observes its temperature, texture, tenseness or laxness, moistness or dryness, and also looks for tenderness and crepitation. Turgor is the degree to which tissue spaces, particularly in the skin and subcutaneous tissues, are filled with extracellular fluid. When a zone of normally lax skin, such as on the abdomen, is gently picked up between thumb and finger and then released, it should flatten out again immediately. Failure to do so (tenting) indicates poor skin turgor, a sign of significant dehydration.

The skin is warm and dry to the touch.

angioedema, angioneurotic edema	*peau d'orange*
turgor, tension, hydration	tenting
brawny edema, induration	hyperelastosis, laxity
hidebound, taut, tense	dry, coarse, rough
clammy, damp, moist, wet	greasy, oily
cold, cool, hot, warm	fibrosis, sclerosis
atrophy	hypertrophy

In evaluating skin color, the examiner considers the intensity and distribution of normal pigment (melanin) and any abnormal coloration, including cyanosis (blueness), erythema (redness), jaundice (yellowness), and bronzing. Localized or generalized loss of pigment is also noted, as well as any tattoos and surgical or traumatic scars. When local or diffuse redness is present, a diascope can be used to distinguish capillary dilatation from other causes. A diascope is a small flat piece of clear glass or plastic, which is pressed firmly against the reddened skin. Blanching (fading of redness) on pressure indicates that redness is probably due to dilatation

color, hue, shade, tinge, tint	
pallor, paleness	ashen, cadaverous, pale, pallid, sallow, waxy
erythema, erythroderma, hyperemia, injection, redness, rubedo, rubor	
a diffuse sunburnlike erythroderma blanching on pressure	angry, beefy red
palmar erythema	malar flush

of skin capillaries. Redness that is due to hemorrhage or abnormal pigmentation will not fade on pressure.

tache cérébrale	flare
cyanosis	nail-bed, peripheral cyanosis
livedo reticularis, marbling, mottling	
ecchymosis, extravasated blood, hematoma, petechiae, purpura	
capillary fragility	Rumpel-Leede test
melanosis, melasma	ephelis, freckle, lentigo
incontinentia pigmenti	bronzing, tanning
café au lait spot	Mongolian spot
albinism, depigmentation, hypopigmentation, leukoderma, vitiligo	
tache bleuâtre	chloasma
chrysoderma, icterus, jaundice	
a large professional tattoo on the lateral aspect of the left arm	
a well-healed traumatic scar	cicatrix, scar, keloid

Although disorders of the skin can produce a seemingly infinite variety of abnormal appearances, the possible range of basic structural changes is limited. These basic **lesions** can be briefly defined as follows:

macule—a zone less than 1 cm in diameter that differs from surrounding skin in color but not in texture or elevation.

petechia—a pinhead-sized red or purple macule due to hemorrhage into the skin.

purpura—a zone of cutaneous hemorrhage larger than a petechia but less than 1 cm in diameter.

ecchymosis—a zone of cutaneous hemorrhage 1 cm or larger in diameter.

telangiectasis—a zone of dilated small blood vessels visible through the skin surface.

papule—a local elevation of skin less than 1 cm in diameter.

nodule—a local elevation 1 cm or more in diameter.

wheal—a small white or red zone of cutaneous edema (a hive).

vesicle—a thin-walled sac containing clear fluid, less than 1 cm in diameter.

bleb (bulla) – a thin-walled sac containing clear fluid, 1 cm or more in diameter (a blister).

pustule—a thin-walled sac containing pus.

cyst—a thick-walled sac containing fluid or semisolid material.

scale—a flake of epidermis shed from the surface.

crust (scab)—an irregular, friable layer of blood, serum, pus, tissue debris, or several of these, adherent at the site of cutaneous injury or inflammation.

erosion (excoriation)—a surface defect in the skin caused by mechanical or inflammatory damage.

fissure—a linear crack in the epidermis.

ulcer—a break in the integrity of the skin surface extending into the dermis.

For Quick Reference

dermatitis
dermatosis
dermis
detritus
diascope
diffuse erythroderma
dome-shaped papule
draining sinus
dyshidrotic eczema
dystrophic nails
ecchymosis (pl. ecchymoses)
ecthyma
eczema, eczematization
ephelis
epidermis
eponychium
erosion (excoriation)
erysipelas
erythema multiforme
erythema nodosum
erythematous halo
erythroderma
eschar
exanthem
exfoliative dermatitis
extravasated blood
exudate
factitial dermatitis
favus
felon
female escutcheon
fibrinous exudate
fibrosis
filiform wart
fissure
fistula
flammeus
floating nails
fluted nails
folliculitis
foreign body
full-thickness burn
fungating
furuncle
furunculosis
gangrene
genital wart
glabrous skin
gouge
granulation tissue
granuloma
guttate
hair follicle
hair shaft
heaped-up border
hematoma
hemorrhage
herpes simplex

For Quick Reference

herpetic whitlow
herpetiform
hippocratic nails
hirsutism
hives
hyperelastosis
hyperemia
hyperhidrosis
hyperkeratosis
hypertrichosis
hypertrophic scar
hypopigmentation
icterus, icteric
imbricated
impetiginization
impetigo
incised wound
incontinentia pigmenti
indurated, induration
intertrigo
iris lesion
Janeway spots
jaundice
keloid scar
keratin plug
keratosis
kerion
kissing ulcer
Koebner phenomenon
koilonychia
lanugo
lentigo
leukoderma
leukonychia
lichenification
linear distribution of lesions
lipoma
livedo reticularis
lupus erythematosus
maceration
macule
maculopapular
malar flush
male escutcheon
male pattern baldness
melanin
melanosis
melasma
milaria
molluscum contagiosum
Mongolian spot
morbilliform
mottling
mucocutaneous
nail plate
nasolabial crease
necrosis
nevus araneus

scar (cicatrix)—a zone of fibrous tissue formed to repair a defect due to injury or disease.

keloid—a hypertrophic, irregular, often pigmented scar.

lichenification—thickening and coarsening of skin, sometimes with pigment change, due to chronic irritation, most often scratching by the subject.

Equally important in diagnosis is the pattern or distribution of lesions—whether diffuse, linear, clustered, confluent, limited to certain anatomic regions, or showing an obvious outline, such as the area covered by an article of clothing or jewelry.

erythematous halo

maculopapular   papulosquamous

papilloma   molluscum contagiosum

xanthelasma, xanthoma

umbilicated   fungating   vegetation

verruca, wart, condyloma acuminatum

wart: filiform, genital, pedunculated, periungual, plantar, sessile, venereal

vesiculobullous   pemphigoid

herpes simplex, zoster   shingles   herpetiform, zosteriform

pimple, abscess, furuncle, pyoderma   pyogenic granuloma

blemish, zit, comedo

wheal and flare   hives, urticaria

exfoliation, exfoliative dermatitis   branny, castlike desquamation

debris, detritus, eschar, scutulum   favus, kerion

scratch marks   ulcer   crater   sloughing

ulcer: deep, irregular, punched-out, shallow, rodent, round

decubitus ulcer, bedsore   contact, kissing ulcer   chancre

a large round ulcer with a heaped-up, indurated border and shaggy, fibrinous exudate adherent to the base

fistula, sinus tract   foreign body

keloid   hypertrophic scar

maceration

stretch marks, striae   proud flesh, granulation tissue

callus, callosity   cellulitis

cherry, spider, strawberry angioma   cavernous hemangioma

vascular lake, nevus, spider   port wine stain   nevus araneus, flammeus

telangiectasis   rubber bleb nevus

Malignant tumors of the skin are not uncommon in older persons, particularly on sun-exposed parts of the body such as the face and neck. In addition, a very small percentage of pigmented lesions in younger persons prove to be highly malignant melanomas. For these reasons all skin tumors and pigmented lesions are subjected to critical scrutiny.

solar, senile keratosis

acuminate, filiform, fungating, papillomatous, pedunculated, sessile

a pigmented nevus with notched and scalloped borders and varying shades and speckles of tan, brown, black, and blue

a bright red, dome-shaped papule on the right cheek just lateral to the nasolabial crease

a pearly-gray papule on the right ala nasi with a central dell and surrounding telangiectasis

Oil and sweat glands, hair, and nails are known as dermal appendages because they arise in or from skin tissue. Abnormalities of sweating may have neural or endocrine origins. Nail disorders are seldom of more than local significance but occasionally reflect systemic disease. Excessive hair growth, abnormal hair loss, and discoloration or deformation of hair shafts may also indicate either local or general disease. Abnormalities of the distribution of body hair can indicate chromosomal or gonadal disorders.

dermal appendages   seborrheic dermatitis

sweat glands, sudoriferous glands   sebum, oil   pilosebaceous unit

anhidrosis, hyperhidrosis   milaria, (prickly) heat rash

dyshidrotic eczema, pompholyx   hair follicle, shaft

alopecia, baldness, calvities   male pattern baldness   temporal recession

canities, graying, poliosis **of the hair**   piebald forelock

hairiness, hirsuties, hirsutism, hypertrichosis   lanugo

male, female escutcheon   pediculosis, phthiriasis   nits

nail plate   nail fold, eponychium   twenty-nail involvement

onycholysis, onychogryphosis, onychophytosis   Beau lines

leukonychia, koilonychia, paronychia   splinter hemorrhage

nails: concave drumstick, dystrophic, floating, fluted, hippocratic, parrot-beak, pitted, serpent-head

subungual hematoma

In most cases of trauma, the skin is affected in some way. Open injuries are described as abrasions (due to scraping away of the skin surface), incised wounds (due to sharp, bladelike objects), punctures, and lacerations (bursting of skin due to blunt trauma). Closed injuries are generally contusions, sometimes with formation of a hematoma (a pocket of leaked blood within tissue). Burns may be described as partial- or full-thickness burns, or graded: first degree, erythema; second degree, blistering; third degree, charring.

open wound   abrasion, gouge, scrape, scratch

tissue defect

incised wound, cut   puncture

For Quick Reference

seropurulent drainage
serosanguineous drainage
serous drainage
serpent-head nails
serpiginous
sessile wart
shaggy exudate
shallow ulcer
shingles
silvery scales
sinus tract
skin warm and dry
sloughing
solar keratosis
speckles of tan, brown, black, and blue
spider angioma
splinter hemorrhage
stasis dermatitis
stellate laceration
stratum corneum
strawberry angioma
streaks and clusters
stretch marks
striae
subcutaneous tissue
subungual hematoma
sudoriferous glands
sweat glands
tache bleuâtre
tache cérébrale
target lesion
telangiectasis
temporal recession
tenting
tinea
tissue defect
tophus
traumatic scar
turgor
twenty-nail involvement
umbilicated
urticaria
vascular lake
vegetation
venereal wart
verruca
vesicle
vesiculobullous
violaceous plaque
vitiligo
wheal
wheal and flare
whitlow
xanthelasma
xanthoma
zit
zoster
zosteriform

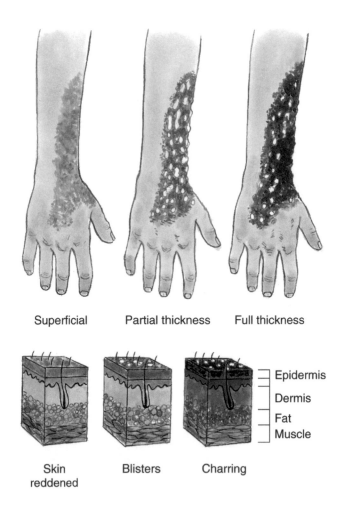

Superficial   Partial thickness   Full thickness

Epidermis
Dermis
Fat
Muscle

Skin reddened   Blisters   Charring

laceration	stellate, bursting-type laceration
closed wound	bruise, contusion
burn, scald	frostbite, chilblain, pernio
full-thickness, partial-thickness burn	

Infections of the skin and immediately subjacent soft tissues are common, resulting usually from penetrating injury but occasionally from invasion of diseased tissue by opportunistic bacteria. The examiner notes the pattern of lesions, the degree of inflammation, and any pus or exudate present.

secondary infection	pyoderma, impetigo, ecthyma
carbuncle, furuncle	furunculosis
cellulitis, erysipelas	pyogenic granuloma
festering, pus, pyogenic, suppuration	oozing, weeping, seeping, draining
drainage: caseous, cheesy, curdy, purulent, sanious, serosanguineous, seropurulent, serous	
folliculitis	felon, paronychia, whitlow herpetic whitlow

Exercises for Chapter 17

Review and Summarize

A. Multiple Choice

___ 1. Which of the following is the correct definition for *excoriation*?
   a. A zone of dilated small blood vessels visible through the skin surface.
   b. A linear crack in the epidermis.
   c. A flake of epidermis.
   d. A surface defect in the skin often caused by scratching.

___ 2. Which of the following is a dermal appendage?
   a. Sweat glands.
   b. Tumor.
   c. Corium.
   d. Epidermis.

___ 3. Erythema of the skin appears
   a. Blue.
   b. Red.
   c. Yellow.
   d. Orange.

___ 4. Poor skin turgor is a sign of significant
   a. Dehydration.
   b. Pigmentation.
   c. Fever.
   d. Infection.

___ 5. A zone of fibrous tissue formed to repair a skin injury is known as a(n)
   a. Ulcer.
   b. Scab.
   c. Scar.
   d. Bleb.

B. Fill in the Blank

1. A pinhead-sized red or purple macule due to hemorrhage into the skin is known as a(n) _____.

2. Scraping away of skin on the surface is known as a(n) _____.

C. Short Answer

1. Describe first-degree, second-degree, and third-degree burns.

_____

_____

_____

_____

2. How is a keloid different from a regular scar?

_____

_____

3. Write a short definition of the following terms. If you can, condense the definition into just a few words or a single synonym that you feel more comfortable with.

a. Cutis _____

b. Ephelis _____

c. Glabrous_____

d. Keratosis _____

e. Fistula_____

f. Necrosis _____

g. Tophus _____

h. Lipoma _____

i. Angioedema _____

j. Turgor_____

k. Tenting _____

l. Fibrosis_____

m. Hypertrophy _____

n. Erythema _____

o. Cyanosis_____

p. Mottling _____

Pause and Reflect

Draw a mind map for this chapter using the skin as the center circle and filling in secondary circles with the dermal appendages: oil and sweat glands, hair, and nails. Working only with the terms described in the text, add conditions and findings to your mind map, connecting them directly to the skin or to the secondary appendages.

Relate and Remember

Take a sheet of paper and draw lines to create four columns, labeled A through D. List five important things to remember about the chapter. Put these in column A. In column B, next to each of the items to remember, write the name of an object that might help you to remember the fact. In column C, write the name of a place that might help you to remember the fact. In column D, write a description of a visual image with which you can associate the fact in column A.

Collaborate and Share

In groups of 3 to 5 students, write 1 to 3 questions about the chapter on separate pieces of paper and crumple them into "snowballs." The instructor then mixes up the "snowballs" and throws them out to the groups, who then answer and discuss the questions within their group. If you get your own question back, return it to the instructor.

Explain and Learn

Using colored dots (or a drawn dot or star), mark what you feel is the most important point or line in each paragraph. If you feel there are multiple important points, rate them and mark the most important with, for example, a red dot, a secondary point with a yellow dot, and the least important point with a green dot. Once you have done this, share your findings with two or three classmates near you. Do you all agree? Discuss any differences of opinion and justify your final decisions.

Relax and Play

1. On a 3" x 5" card, write a question pertaining to the chapter and give the card to your instructor. The instructor tosses a koosh ball, small stuffed animal, net bath sponge, or some other soft object, at random to an individual student. When the object is tossed to you, answer the question the instructor reads from one of the cards.

2. Fold a blank piece of paper in half three times so that when unfolded there are eight squares. Write one thing you learned in each square. Move around the room, asking other students to define or explain an item on your sheet. That student then signs the square. The student who gets all eight squares signed first wins.

Generalize and Apply

In the paragraph describing the evaluation of skin color, *cyanosis* is defined as blueness, *erythema* as redness, and *jaundice* as yellowness. Other colors can be used to describe skin lesions. Locate as many terms describing skin color as you can, using the list of terms in this chapter and any other resources. Where possible, show both the medical and lay terms for each color.

_____

_____

_____

_____

_____

_____

_____

Compare and Contrast

1. Confusion between the similar-sounding adjectives *purpuric* and *pruritic* often leads to transcription errors. Using a medical dictionary and your textbooks, determine the similarities and differences in the origins of these terms (etymology) and in their meaning and usage.

_____

_____

_____

_____

2. *Scar* and *eschar* are also frequently confused. Research these terms as you did for the question above and propose a method by which you would differentiate between these terms while transcribing.

_____

_____

_____

_____

Extrapolate and Project

A compromised immune system, such as in patients with acquired immunodeficiency syndrome, leads to opportunistic infections, many of which manifest in the skin. Where would you find information about these conditions? Using the sources you identified, locate the names of these conditions and describe the skin symptoms that accompany them.

_____

_____

_____

_____

_____

_____

18

Examination of the Head, Face, and Neck

The physician usually begins the examination with the head and face, since they are normally uncovered by clothing and are the parts at which one naturally looks first in viewing or studying another person. The examiner notes the size, shape, and symmetry of the skull, palpating for swellings, lumps, or tenderness. Deformities of the skull can be congenital (as a feature of many inherited deforming syndromes) or acquired (as in acromegaly and Paget disease).

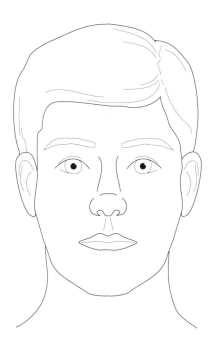

Head: Normocephalic.

The head is symmetrical and normally developed, without exostoses or traumatic lesions.

skull, cranium, calvaria   lambdoid crest   occiput

frontal, parietal, occipital, temporal   supraorbital ridge

inion, external occipital protuberance   asterion, nasion, pterion

forehead   glabella   temple   coronal, sagittal suture

mastoid process   nuchal muscles

brachycephalic, dolichocephalic

macrocephaly   microcephaly   *cracked-pot note*

Paget disease   craniotabes

cranial bosses   cephalhematoma, *goose-egg*

The amount, distribution, texture, and color of scalp hair are observed, as well as the pattern of any hair loss. The scalp is inspected for scaling, dermatitis, signs of acute or past trauma, and other lesions. Any tremors or involuntary movements of the head are noted.

alopecia, baldness, calvities   alopecia areata, generalisata, totalis

male-pattern baldness   temporal recession   widow's peak

anagen, telogen effluvium

canities, graying, poliosis   piebald forelock

dandruff, scaling   tinea capitis

favus, kerion   Battle sign

tremor, twitch   *bishop's nod*, Musset sign

A mere glance at the **face** will usually suffice to tell the examiner whether the subject is alert or somnolent, anxious or apathetic, angry or euphoric. The face not only registers the patient's current emotional state but often reflects systemic

Learning Objectives

After careful study of this chapter, you should be able to:

Name conditions that produce changes in facial features.

Describe conditions for which facial swelling may be diagnostic.

Identify terminology that characterizes cutaneous eruptions and changes in skin color.

Discuss conditions affecting athe neck.

Describe the examination of the external jugular veins.

For Quick Reference

disease as well. Parkinsonism, myxedema, acromegaly, myasthenia gravis, allergic rhinitis, and Cushing syndrome each produce characteristic changes in facial features.

---

face, facies   mandible   maxilla   zygoma

face (facies): adenoid, allergic, cushingoid, hippocratic, leonine, masklike, mongoloid, *moon*, parkinsonian, wizened, wrinkled

hollow, sunken cheeks   *bouche de tapir*   *alar flaring*

ashen, cadaverous, pale, pallid, sallow, waxy   deathly pallor

beefy red, beet red, florid, flushed, plethoric   malar flush

circumoral flush, circumoral pallor   melasma

cyanotic, leaden, livid

chrysoderma, icterus, jaundice

periorbital ecchymosis   *raccoon eyes*   *allergic shiners*

Generalized changes in skin color (pallor, flushing, cyanosis, jaundice, abnormal pigmentation) are apt to be noted first in the face because it is uncovered by clothing and seen first. Color changes may, however, be largely confined to the face, as with the circumoral pallor of scarlatina and the malar flush of tuberculosis.

Facial configuration and symmetry can be distorted by various congenital syndromes. Paralysis due to peripheral neuropathy (Bell palsy) or stroke can also cause facial asymmetry, as a result of impaired mobility of one part of the face. The examiner may instruct the patient to perform various movements such as wrinkling the forehead, showing the teeth, and pursing the lips to whistle, in order to test for facial muscle weakness or paralysis.

---

platybasia   upturned nose with a long philtrum

ocular hypertelorism, hypotelorism   facial hemiatrophy

pursed-lip breathing   rictus

Bell palsy   bulbar, pseudobulbar palsy

tic, twitch   habit spasm

tetany   risus sardonicus   Chvostek sign

Cutaneous eruptions may be largely confined to the face (acne, rosacea, the malar rash of lupus erythematosus) or may appear there as part of a general exanthem (varicella). The lips are subject to conditions that seldom affect other parts of the skin. Masses or cutaneous nodules are carefully evaluated for signs of malignancy. The examiner notes the presence and character of any facial hair. A mustache or beard may be worn to conceal surgical or traumatic scars or other lesions; these must be looked for.

---

acne (vulgaris)   cystic acne   (acne) rosacea   pitting, scarring

butterfly   *eruption, erythema, rash*   telangiectasia, telangiectases

cheiloschisis, cleft lip, harelip

cheilitis, cheilosis   angular cheilitis   rhagades
herpes labialis, simplex   perlèche
thinning of the outer thirds of the eyebrows
Dennie sign, Morgan lines

Subtle degrees of swelling may not be apparent if the examiner has had no previous acquaintance with the patient. Facial swelling can be diffuse or can affect certain areas more than others—the eyelids in infectious mononucleosis, the cheeks in Cushing syndrome, the lips in angioneurotic edema. Swelling over a paranasal sinus can indicate underlying infection. Swelling of the parotid gland occurs in mumps and obstruction of a salivary duct, but may also represent a tumor. The physician carefully palpates any facial swelling or mass to assess its consistency, tenderness, and other significant features.

parotid gland   facial edema, fullness, puffiness, swelling

Pain in the lower **jaw** or difficulty in chewing or speaking will prompt an assessment of the mandible, the temporomandibular joints, and the muscles of mastication for mobility, spasm, swelling, crepitus, or tenderness.

masseter   temporalis   muscles of mastication
micrognathia   prognathism
trismus   TMJ (temporomandibular joint)

The **neck** is not simply a column for supporting the head. Through it pass all nerve connections between brain and body, all inspired oxygen and exhaled carbon dioxide, all swallowed food and drink, and all blood supply to the brain, which consumes 25 percent of the body's oxygen intake. Because subtle abnormalities of the neck can herald life-threatening developments, the region is carefully assessed.

Neck: The neck is supple without palpable masses or venous distention.

The neck is subject to many musculoskeletal injuries and disorders, some of which can affect its configuration and mobility in obvious ways. The examiner tests neck mobility by gently grasping the subject's head and putting it through a range of movements, noting any restrictions due to joint stiffness, muscle spasm, or pain.

dewlap   nuchal rigidity
(spastic) torticollis, wryneck   Brudzinski sign
sternocleidomastoid muscle   hyoid bone   thyroid, cricoid cartilage
left, right lobe of thyroid   thyroid isthmus

For Quick Reference

facial edema
facial hemiatrophy
facial puffiness
favus
glabella
goose-egg
habit spasm
harelip
hepatojugular reflux
herpes labialis
herpes simplex
hippocratic face (facies)
hollow cheeks
hyoid bone
icterus
jaundice
jugular venous pulses
jugulodigastric (lymph) nodes
kerion
lambdoid crest
leonine face (facies)
lymph glands
lymph nodes
lymphadenopathy
macromegaly
malar flush of tuberculosis
male-pattern baldness
masseter
masklike face (facies)
mastoid process
matted nodes
melasma
microcephaly
micrognathia
mongoloid face (facies)
moon face (facies)
Morgan lines
multinodular goiter
muscles of mastication
Musset sign
myasthenia gravis
myxedema
nasion
normocephalic
nuchal muscle
nuchal rigidity
occiput
ocular hypertelorism
ocular hypotelorism
Paget disease
parkinsonian face (facies)
parotid gland
periorbital ecchymosis
peripheral neuropathy
perlèche
philtrum
piebald forelock
pitting

For Quick Reference

platybasia
plethoric
poliosis
postauricular (lymph) nodes
preauricular (lymph) nodes
prognathism
pseudobulbar palsy
pterion
pursed-lip breathing
raccoon eyes
rhagades
rictus
risus sardonicus
sagittal suture
scarring
sentinel node
shotty nodes
sternocleidomastoid muscle
submandibular (lymph) nodes
submental (lymph) nodes
suboccipital (lymph) nodes
sunken cheeks
supraclavicular (lymph) nodes
supraorbital ridge
telangiectasia (pl. telangiectases)
telogen effluvium
temporal recession
temporalis
tetany
thyroglossal duct cyst
thyroid cartilage
thyroid isthmus
thyroid nodule
tinea capitis
TMJ (temporomandibular joint)
torticollis
tracheal deviation
tracheal tug
tremor
trismus
Troisier node
twitch
uninodular goiter
Virchow node
widow's peak
wizened face (facies)
wrinkled face (facies)
wryneck

Any swellings or masses are palpated for size, shape, consistency, mobility, pulsatility, and tenderness. Additionally, the entire neck is felt for enlarged lymph nodes, which may appear in any of several locations. Each anatomic group of nodes "drains" (receives lymphatic channels from) a specific region of the head, face, neck, or thorax. The thyroid gland is felt and its size and consistency assessed. For this examination the physician may ask the patient to swallow in order to move the gland up and down under the palpating fingers. The larynx and the uppermost part of the trachea are also felt and any lesions or lateral deviation noted.

branchial cleft cyst   thyroglossal duct cyst

anterior, posterior cervical lymphadenopathy

lymph glands, lymph nodes, nodes

(lymph) nodes: jugulodigastric, submandibular, submental, suboccipital, supra-clavicular, preauricular, postauricular

nodes: shotty, matted, discrete   Virchow, Troisier node   *sentinel node*

Delphian nodes

The thyroid is diffusely enlarged, smooth, and nontender.

thyroid nodule   diffuse, multinodular, uninodular goiter

tracheal deviation   *tracheal tug*

The pulsations of the **carotid arteries** are gently palpated and compared. The physician applies a stethoscope over each carotid in turn to listen for bruits—harsh sounds synchronous with the pulse, caused by passage of blood through a vessel narrowed by arteriosclerosis.

Carotid pulses are full and equal; no carotid bruits are heard.
carotid sinus massage

The **external jugular veins** at the sides of the neck are normally not distended with blood when one is in an upright position, but can be seen to be filled with blood in the recumbent position. The physician can judge the patient's venous pressure by noting the height to which the upper body must be raised from the horizontal before the external jugular veins are no longer visibly distended. Increased venous pressure, which occurs in cardiac failure, may cause the jugular veins to remain filled even in the erect position. Pressure over the liver may cause the level of blood in the external jugular veins to rise in congestive heart failure (hepato-jugular reflux). The internal jugular veins are not visible, but they can impart faint pulsations to the soft tissues of the neck that are coordinated in a complex way with cardiac function.

The external jugulars are visibly distended at 45°.
Neck veins are elevated to the angle of the jaw at 90°.
Jugular venous pulses are seen at 60° elevation.
a/c/v wave

Exercises for Chapter 18

Review and Summarize

A. Multiple Choice

____ 1. A bruit is
   a. A swelling in the neck.
   b. A harsh sound in an artery.
   c. An involuntary movement of the head and neck.
   d. A large discolored area on the head or neck.

____ 2. The brain consumes what percent of the body's oxygen intake?
   a. 15%.
   b. 20%.
   c. 25%.
   d. 30%.

____ 3. Hepatojugular reflux is often diagnostic of
   a. Kidney failure.
   b. Neck vein collapse.
   c. Liver damage.
   d. Congestive heart failure.

B. Fill in the Blank

1. Deformities of the skull can be either acquired or _____.

2. A skin nodule or mass is carefully evaluated for signs of _____.

3. The _____ arteries in the neck may be checked for blockage with a stethoscope.

C. Short Answer

1. Why is the observation of facial features so important upon examination of the head, face, and neck?

_____

_____

2. List the conditions that might restrict neck motion.

_____

_____

3. Describe the functions of the neck.

_____

_____

_____

_____

_____

4. Write a short definition of the following terms. If you can, condense the definition into just a few words or a single synonym that you feel more comfortable with.

a. Torticollis _____

b. Occiput _____

c. Parietal _____

d. Glabella _____

e. Brachycephalic _____

f. Boss _____

g. Alopecia _____

h. Poliosis _____

i. Tremor _____

j. Zygoma _____

k. Wizened _____

l. Pallid _____

m. Platybasia _____

n. Perlèche _____

o. Mastication _____

p. Myxedema _____

Pause and Reflect

Type or handwrite below the physical examination of your own head, face, and neck using the criteria described in this chapter. Be sure to indicate pertinent negatives as well as positive findings.

_____

_____

_____

_____

_____

_____

Relate and Remember

Think of a metaphor that completes this statement: The head, face, or neck (choose one) is like a _____ _____. Use a visual or a verbal metaphor. You may fill in the blank with the name of an object or draw (or cut out of a magazine) a picture representing one or more important points. Explain your choice.

_____

_____

_____

_____

_____

_____

_____

Collaborate and Share

Label a blank sheet of paper with your name at the top and write a question requiring a short answer (less than a sentence) related to this chapter. Pass this paper to the student on your right, who will answer the question and then add a question of his or her own, as you answer the question on the paper received from the student on your left. Each sheet moves around the room until everyone has had a turn with every paper and you end up with the paper with your name at the top. Choose the best question(s) and answer(s) from your page to read aloud when called upon by your instructor.

Explain and Learn

List below everything you know about this chapter. As a group, pick 1 to 3 most important points and share with the class.

_____

_____

_____

_____

_____

_____

Relax and Play

1. After reviewing the chapter as a class or in small groups, the instructor will announce "Go," and individual class members will "pop up" and call out one important fact learned, already known, or remembered about a topic or section in this chapter.

2. Select 10 to 20 words or phrases from the word list in this chapter and create a word search puzzle. Rather than list the words you've chosen, however, list the definitions as clues. Copy the puzzle to share with the rest of the class. Students must first determine which word goes with the definition before finding it in the puzzle.

Generalize and Apply

Write a letter to your teacher describing something you learned in this chapter and how you think this information will help you in your future career.

_____

_____

_____

_____

_____

_____

Compare and Contrast

What's the difference between *reflux* and *reflex*? Are their similarities in their usage? Give examples of their usage in the head, face, and neck exam.

_____

_____

_____

Extrapolate and Project

John Merrick, the "Elephant Man," suffered from a disfiguring disorder most visible on his head and neck for which many diagnoses have been proposed, including neurofibromatosis and, more recently, Proteus syndrome. Obtain a photo of John Merrick from a library book or encyclopedia (or rent the video of "The Elephant Man") and study the appearance of his head and neck. Without consulting any published research, propose your own explanation for his disfigurement.

_____

_____

_____

_____

_____

_____

_____

_____

_____

_____

_____

_____

19

Examination of the Eyes

The eyes are subject to many acute and chronic diseases, some of which can threaten vision. Moreover, the eyes register or reflect many systemic disorders such as arteriosclerosis, diabetes, thyrotoxicosis, and diseases of the nervous system. Hence they deserve attentive examination. Unless some historical point has drawn particular attention to one or both eyes, the physician's evaluation will usually be limited to an inspection of the lids and lashes and the parts of the eye exposed between them, a test of the pupillary light reflexes, a rough check of ocular movements and visual fields, and an inspection of the ocular fundi. A test of vision is often included. All of these procedures can be performed quickly and easily with standard equipment, but several of them require the cooperation of the patient.

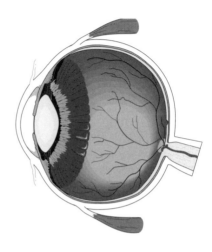

glass eye, ocular prosthesis   presently wearing contact lenses

right eye (OD)   left eye (OS)   both eyes (OU)

inner, nasal canthus   outer, temporal canthus

Normally the patient sits upright for the eye examination, if possible. The orbital margins are inspected for swelling or ecchymosis, and may be palpated for tenderness if any clue to recent trauma is noted. The lids are observed for evidence of deformity, swelling, discoloration, masses, crusting, or disorders of the tear glands and ducts. Bulging or protrusion of one or both eyes (exophthalmos) can result from hyperthyroidism or orbital disease.

conjunctiva   cornea   globe   limbus   meibomian gland
The left eye is swollen nearly shut and the lids are deeply discolored.
Palpation of the orbital rim discloses no skeletal tenderness or crepitus.
periorbital ecchymosis, black eye, *raccoon eye(s)*   exophthalmos
thinning of the lateral thirds of the eyebrows
enophthalmos, hollow, sunken eyes
narrowing of the palpebral fissures   lagophthalmos   symblepharon
ptosis, lid lag, epicanthal folds, ectropion, entropion
(marginal) blepharitis, crusting of the lids, pediculosis of the lashes
petechiae of the palpebral conjunctiva   xanthelasma
stye, hordeolum, pustule   dacryoadenitis, dacryocystitis
chalazion, meibomian cyst, tarsal cyst   decreased blinking

Learning Objectives

After careful study of this chapter, you should be able to:

List the major components of a routine eye exam.

Classify eye exam findings by the ocular structures they describe.

Describe the method by which a lesion on the inner eyelid can be detected.

Explain pupillary light reflex testing.

Describe the method by which visual fields are assessed.

Name the principal structures of the optic fundus and describe the role of the ophthalmoscope in their examination.

Identify systemic conditions that can be diagnosed by examination of the eye.

For Quick Reference

The **anterior chamber** of the eye—the part in front of the pupil—is easily studied with the help of a hand lamp. The physician looks for opacities in the cornea and anterior chamber, abnormalities of the iris, and irregularities in the shape of the pupil, incidentally observing whether the pupil constricts when light is shown directly into the eye. This procedure also serves as a test for photophobia (abnormal sensitivity to light). A check of the accommodation reflex may also be made by asking the patient to look at a distant object and noting whether the pupils constrict. Astigmatism, a warping of the cornea out of its expected spherical form, can sometimes be detected by noting distortion in the reflection of some regularly shaped object on the cornea, but is more precisely determined by vision testing with refracting lenses designed for the purpose which only an ophthalmologist would normally have on hand. The location of a lesion of the cornea or iris is indicated by the hour position to which it would be nearest if the eye were a clock dial (e.g., 5 o'clock).

anterior segment, anterior chamber   hypopyon, hyphema

corneal opacity, keratoconus, keratitis   astigmatism

dewy, grainy, steamy cornea   keratoconjunctivitis   arcus senilis, circus senilis

band keratopathy   Kayser-Fleischer ring   Brushfield spots

The pupils are round, regular, and equal and react to light and accommodation.

anisocoria, iridonesis, tremulous iris   hippus

coloboma (iridis)   *status post* iridectomy for glaucoma   iris bombé

Direct and consensual light reflexes are intact.

Marcus Gunn pupil   Argyll Robertson pupil

Adie pupil   Horner syndrome

The pupils are dilated and fixed. The corneal reflex is absent.

blown pupil   ophthalmoplegia   iritis, iridocyclitis, uveitis

an embedded foreign body at 3 o'clock   aphakia

Abnormalities of the white of the eye can be due to discoloration or disease of the **sclera** or of the overlying **conjunctiva**, usually the latter. Mild or early jaundice is typically more evident in the scleras than in the skin. Conjunctival swelling and discharge or lacrimation (excessive tearing) are noted, as well as the degree and

The scleras are deeply icteric, jaundiced.   blue scleras

episcleritis, pterygium, pinguecula   anterior staphyloma

chemosis, edema, swelling of the conjunctiva   Bitot spots

ciliary injection, limbal flush   *cobblestoning* of the palpebral conjunctiva

conjunctival injection, hyperemia, erythema, congestion, redness

conjunctivitis: allergic, phlyctenular, vernal, epidemic, purulent

a small (sub)conjunctival hemorrhage at the inner canthus of the left eye

profuse lacrimation, watery   epiphora   xerophthalmia

copious mucopurulent discharge

distribution of any redness. Very thin scleras, such as occur in some connective tissue disorders, appear blue.

Imbalance of the **extraocular muscles** may or may not be readily apparent. Imbalances are called tropias when the eyes cannot be made to look in the same direction, phorias when there is a tendency to deviation that the patient habitually controls so as not to see double. Even a slight degree of tropia can sometimes be detected by observing whether the reflections of a handheld lamp appear at corresponding points on the two corneas. Tropias and phorias can also be demonstrated with the cover test. The patient gazes steadily at a distant object and the examiner covers first one eye and then the other, noting whether one or both eyes swing into a different position immediately after being uncovered. This test depends on intact vision in both eyes; however, in an uncorrected tropia, vision is eventually lost in one eye.

> esophoria, esotropia, convergent strabismus, cross-eyedness
>
> comitant strabismus, conjugate deviation   cover test
>
> medial, nasal deviation   lateral, temporal deviation
>
> horizontal, vertical, rotatory nystagmus
>
> horizontal nystagmus with the quick, fast component to the right
>
> Eyes: No gross abnormalities. Pupils constricted.
>
> Eyes: Examination of the eyes reveals pupils that react to light in a normal manner. The optic fundi are normal. His extraocular motions are normal, and there is no nystagmus.

The physician tests the integrity of the extraocular muscles (the voluntary muscles, six for each eye, that control the direction of gaze) by having the examinee follow the movements of a handheld object such as a lamp while holding the head immobile. Abnormalities of ocular movement can be due to disease or injury of the brain or of the third, fourth, or sixth cranial nerve on either side, or to orbital disease or injury affecting one or more of the extraocular muscles.

> medial, lateral, superior, inferior rectus muscle   superior, inferior oblique
>
> third cranial nerve, oculomotor nerve   fourth cranial nerve, trochlear nerve
>
> sixth cranial nerve, abducens nerve
>
> right sixth nerve palsy   oculomotor nerve palsy
>
> EOMs (extraocular muscles) are normal.
>
> EOMI (extraocular muscles intact).
>
> The pupils respond to light and accommodation. The extraocular muscles are hard to test.
>
> Extraocular muscles were intact. The pupils are equal, round, and reactive to light.

The **visual field** of an eye is that part of the space before it that it can see while held motionless. Abnormalities of visual field, which can be caused by retinal or neural disease or injury, represent partial loss of vision in the form of blind spots (scotomata) or narrowed range of vision. Visual fields can be roughly tested by the confrontation method. The subject is instructed to gaze at the examiner's nose

For Quick Reference

crossing phenomena
crusting of lids
dacryoadenitis
dacryocystitis
dead-white disk
dendritic keratitis
dewy cornea
diabetic retinopathy
direct light reflexes
discolored lids
disk (disc)
drusen
ectropion
edema of the conjunctiva
embedded foreign body
emmetropia
enophthalmos
entropion
epicanthal folds
epidemic conjunctivitis
epiphora
episcleritis
erythema
esophoria
esotropia
exophthalmos
exudates
eye grounds
farsightedness
flame hemorrhages
fluorescein examination
focal and diffuse arteriolar narrowing
foreign body
fovea (centralis)
fundus (pl. fundi)
glass eye
globe
grade III Keith-Wagener (KW) changes
grainy cornea
hard exudates
hemorrhages
herpetic keratitis
hippus
hollow eyes
homonymous hemianopsia
hordeolum
Horner syndrome
humping
hyperemia
hypermetropia
hypertensive retinopathy
hyphema
hypopyon
icteric sclerae
impaired peripheral vision
inferior rectus muscle
inferior oblique muscle
iridocyclitis

For Quick Reference

while first one eye and then the other is covered. The examiner moves a finger or a light from the side and then from above and below into the subject's range of vision and the subject reports when the object first becomes visible. If the examiner in turn gazes at the subject's nose (and if the examiner's own visual fields are normal), both should see the object at the same time. More elaborate equipment is needed for more precise mapping of visual fields.

The **optic fundus** is the portion of the interior of the eye that can be seen by an examiner looking through the pupil with an ophthalmoscope, a handheld instrument with a light source and a set of magnifying lenses that can be quickly changed. The principal features of the fundus are the retina, the optic disk or nerve head, and branches of the central retinal artery and vein. Retinal and optic nerve disease, as well as the effects of systemic conditions such as diabetes, arteriosclerosis, and hypertension, are readily observed in the fundus, provided that the examiner's view is not blocked by an opaque lens (cataract) or a hemorrhage or foreign body within the eye.

The examiner adjusts the instrument to compensate for visual deficit (refractive error) in the subject's eye. Since the strength (in diopters) of the lens being used can be read from a scale on the ophthalmoscope, this examination serves as a rough measure of visual acuity. Sizes and distances in the fundus can be measured by comparison with the diameter of the disk. Edema of the disk (choked disk) is measured by the difference between lens settings needed to focus on the disk and on the rest of the fundus. If the pupil is very small it may be dilated with drops in preparation for ophthalmoscopic examination.

> The patient's visual acuity is 20/50 in the right eye. She has visual acuity in the left eye of counting fingers on the basis of aphakia and a pupillary membrane with updrawn pupil. Her optic discs have a cup:disc ratio of 0.34 in each eye and the peripheral retinas are within normal limits.
>
> Eye examination shows best vision of 20/50+ in the right eye and 20/200 in the left. Pupils and extraocular motility are normal. Intraocular pressures are 18. Slit-lamp exam shows the eyelids in good position with weakness of the orbicularis and facial muscles. There is a clear corneal epithelium and the normal pseudophakia of the right eye and a dense nuclear cataract on the left. Fundus examination in each eye is normal.

Vision testing is usually performed with the familiar Snellen wall chart for far vision and a set of Jaeger test types for near vision. The subject reads the lowest (smallest) row of letters that are legible on the wall chart at a distance of 20 feet, and this performance is expressed as a fraction of normal. Thus 20/20 vision indicates normal far visual acuity, while 20/40 means that, at a distance of 20 feet, the subject can see no letters smaller than those that a normal person can see at 40 feet.

For near vision a card bearing a few lines of print in a standard type is held as close to one eye as possible and gradually moved away from it. The examiner notes the distance from the eye at which the subject is first able to read the print and the distance beyond which it can no longer be read. For more precise measurement of near vision, the card may contain various sizes of type. Far and near vision testing

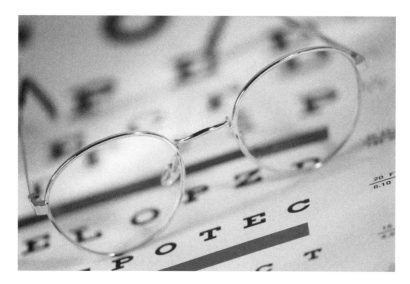

is generally performed on each eye separately and on both eyes together. A subject who wears glasses is tested both with and without them.

normal vision, emmetropia	amaurosis, blindness
myopia, nearsightedness	hypermetropia, farsightedness
amblyopia presbyopia	
red-green color-blindness	Ishihara pseudoisochromatic plates

Color vision can be tested by a variety of methods. The most sophisticated of these are the Ishihara pseudoisochromatic plates, which make it virtually impossible to feign color-blindness and allow identification of the type of color-blindness that is present.

Certain **other simple diagnostic maneuvers** may be dictated by circumstances. The inner surface of the upper lid can more readily be examined if it is exposed by inversion of the lid over a cotton-tipped applicator. Fluorescein dye can be instilled in the eye and the cornea examined for ulcers or abrasions with a cobalt blue light, which causes minute collections of dye to show up clearly as brilliant yellow-green patches.

Firm palpation of the eyeball through the closed lids (moderately uncomfortable and slightly dangerous) can reveal undue hardness, such as occurs in acute and chronic glaucoma. In some settings, tonometry is a routine part of the examination of persons over 40. More sophisticated and elaborate examinations of the eye belong within the province of the ophthalmologist.

corneal ulcer	dendritic, herpetic keratitis

Examination of the cornea with fluorescein reveals a deep abrasion at 4 o'clock.

There is a deeply embedded foreign body in the center of the left cornea, with a rust ring.

No foreign bodies are noted on the palpebral conjunctiva or on the globe.

Exercises for Chapter 19

Review and Summarize

A. Multiple Choice

___ 1. Exophthalmos may be diagnostic of
    a. Hypertension.
    b. Migraine headache.
    c. Diabetes mellitus.
    d. Thyroid disorder.

___ 2. The sclerae are normally what color?
    a. Blue.
    b. White.
    c. Yellow.
    d. Red.

___ 3. Signs of severe diabetes, arteriosclerosis, and hypertension may be noticeable during what portion of the eye exam?
    a. Fundus examination.
    b. Visual field examination.
    c. Scleral examination.
    d. Extraocular examination.

___ 4. A person with 20/100 vision
    a. Sees at 20 feet what a person with normal eyesight sees at 100 feet.
    b. Sees at 100 feet what a person with normal eyesight sees at 20 feet.
    c. Can see for 20 feet clearly in the left eye.
    d. Can see for 20 feet clearly in the right eye.

B. Fill in the Blank

1. Blind spots in the visual fields are known as _____.

2. Tonometry is routinely used by eye specialists to check for the presence of _____.

3. _____ is a green dye used to detect ulcers or abrasions in the eye.

4. Photophobia is _____ to light.

5. The two types of vision tests are _____ and

    _____.

C. Short Answer

1. Write a short definition of the following terms. If you can, condense the definition into just a few words or a single synonym that you feel more comfortable with.

   a. Opacity _____

   b. Prosthesis _____

   c. Chalazion _____

   d. Lacrimation _____

   e. Nystagmus _____

   f. Myopia _____

   g. Hyperopia _____

   h. Astigmatism _____

   i. Strabismus _____

   j. Accommodation reflex _____

   k. Hemianopsia _____

   l. Presbyopia _____

Pause and Reflect

Think about the last time you or a member of your family had an eye examination. What parts of the exam do you remember? What procedures were used? What pieces of equipment do you recall? Circle anything in the text you remember from your examination. Write down any questions you might have for your ophthalmologist or optometrist at your next exam.

_____

_____

_____

_____

_____

Relate and Remember

Using this diagram of the eye, list 3 to 5 terms for each area that the physician might use to describe the findings in that area.

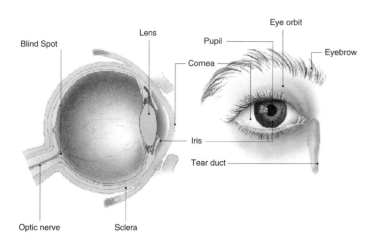

Collaborate and Share

As a group, draw a mind map for the eye exam, listing the tests and diagnostic maneuvers used to examine the eyes in the secondary circles. Before beginning the next layer of circles, trade maps with another group. Then, for the map you now have, fill in the next layer of circles with possible results from these tests and maneuvers. Now trade maps with another group and begin another layer of circles showing one or more diagnoses for each of the positive findings in the third layer.

Explain and Learn

Turn to the person next to you (or behind or in front of you), and share with each other one important piece of information you got from this chapter. Also share how you might use this information in your life or in your work. If you have a question that wasn't answered in the chapter, share that as well. If your partner doesn't have the answer, ask your instructor.

Relax and Play

1. Using the words from the terms list in the chapter, write a poem or song that incorporates the terms in such a way as to reveal their meaning or use. If writing a song, you can use a familiar tune or rap style.

2. With all members of the class standing, choose a term pertaining to the eyes that begins with the letter A and make a statement beginning with this term, such as "Astigmatism is warping of the cornea." The next student makes a statement beginning with the letter B, such as "Blue sclerae can be a symptom of connective tissue disease." Continue through the alphabet, with each student taking the next letter. Anyone who cannot come up with a statement sits down. The winner is the last person standing.

Generalize and Apply

The effects of systemic conditions such as diabetes, arteriosclerosis, and hypertension are readily observed on funduscopic examination. Based on your knowledge of these conditions, speculate on what these findings might include. Compare your assessment with those of your classmates.

_____

_____

_____

_____

_____

_____

Compare and Contrast

 The eye is often compared to a camera. What are the similarities? How are they different? What other comparisons might you make?

_____

_____

_____

_____

_____

_____

Extrapolate and Project

Vision correction is now possible through a variety of surgical procedures. Investigate the types of procedures available and determine which vision deficits can be corrected surgically and which are not amenable to such a procedure. Interview someone who has undergone surgical vision correction. Summarize your findings below.

_____

_____

_____

_____

_____

_____

_____

_____

_____

_____

_____

_____

_____

_____

_____

_____

_____

_____

_____

20

Examination of the Ears

For descriptive purposes the anatomist divides the human ear into three parts. The external ear consists of the pinna and the external auditory meatus or ear canal. The middle ear, or eardrum, is a hollow space within the temporal bone, lined with mucous membrane and communicating via the eustachian (pharyngotympanic or auditory tube) with the nasopharynx. The middle ear is separated from the external ear by the tympanic membrane, and it contains three small bones connected in sequence that transmit sound waves from the tympanic membrane to the cochlea. The inner ear consists of the cochlea, with receptors for the auditory division of the eighth cranial nerve; and the vestibular apparatus, with receptors for the vestibular division of the eighth cranial nerve, which is concerned with equilibrium.

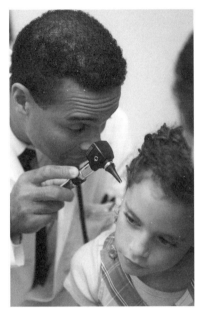

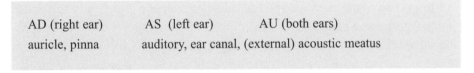

| AD (right ear) | AS (left ear) | AU (both ears) |
| auricle, pinna | auditory, ear canal, (external) acoustic meatus | |

The diagnostician has full access to the external ear, very limited access to the middle ear, and none at all to the inner ear except through testing of hearing and equilibrium.

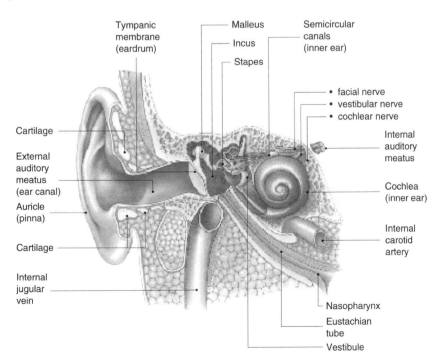

Learning Objectives

After careful study of this chapter, you should be able to:

Identify the three parts of the ear and their components.

Discuss the accessibility of the parts of the ear to external exam.

Describe the methods by which the structures of the external, middle, and internal ear are assessed.

Identify equipment, tests, and findings associated with the ear examination.

Name the two types of hearing loss.

Distinguish between the Rinne and Weber tests.

For Quick Reference

acoustic meatus
AD (right ear)
aerotitis
air-bone gap
anthelix
AS (left ear)
AU (both ears)
audiogram
auditory acuity
auditory canal
auditory discrimination
auditory threshold
auditory tube
auricle
Aztec ear
balance
barotitis
blood in ear
bulging of tympanic membrane
Cagot ear
caloric stimulation
caloric test
cauliflower ear
cholesteatoma
cochlea
conductive hearing loss
cone-shaped specula
darwinian tubercle
deafness
decibels
deeply retracted tympanic membrane
diagonal earlobe creases
discrimination (scrim)
Dix-Hallpike test
ear canal
eardrum
edema
equilibrium
eustachian tube
external ear
exudate in ear
foreign material in ears
gray or opalescent tympanic membrane
grommet
hearing impairment
hearing loss
hearing testing
heel-to-toe walking
helix
hemotympanum
hyperacusis Willisii
impacted cerumen
injected tympanic membrane
injection
inner ear
low-set ears
malfunction of acoustic nerve
manubrium (handle)

Examination of the ear begins with inspection of the pinna for deformity, inflammation, injury, and abnormal masses. The **external ear** is subject to many developmental anomalies, some of which have more than cosmetic importance. Malformations of the external ear occur as part of various inherited syndromes that include faulty development of other structures as well. They may also indicate congenital renal disease. There is a high correlation between diagonal earlobe creases and coronary artery disease in middle-aged and elderly men.

| helix | anthelix | tragus | darwinian tubercle | microtia | low-set ears |

diagonal earlobe creases | Aztec, Cagot, satyr ear

The framework of the pinna is cartilage, a tissue with poor healing potential. Hence severe or repeated trauma to the ear or severe infection can result in permanent deformity. The pinna is a frequent site for the tophi of gout. The earlobe is subject to sebaceous cysts. Piercing of the pinna or earlobe for ornaments sometimes results in infection, hypertrophic scarring, or keloid formation.

cauliflower ear

Inspection of the ear canal and **tympanic membrane** is generally performed with an otoscope, a handheld instrument with a light source, exchangeable cone-shaped specula of various sizes, and a magnifying lens. (A specialist may prefer to use a head mirror or headlamp and handheld specula.) In order to get an adequate view of the tympanic membrane, the examiner must straighten the ear canal by pulling the pinna back and up with one hand while positioning the otoscope with the other. Because otoscopic examination can be performed with one eye only, there is no true depth perception. Accumulated wax (cerumen) or exudate, foreign material, swelling of the ear canal, and inability of the patient to tolerate the insertion of the speculum can all render adequate otoscopic examination difficult or impossible.

Under ideal conditions the examiner inspects the ear canal for injection, edema, impacted cerumen, exudate, blood, and foreign material. The normal tympanic membrane appears gray or opalescent and nearly flat, but with recognizable landmarks. Behind it the manubrium (handle) of the malleus (hammer) can just be seen. Possible abnormalities are injection, bulging, retraction, or perforation of the tympanic membrane; discoloration by blood in the middle ear, which can result from basal skull fracture; a fluid level, bubbles, or both behind the tympanic membrane, indicating serous fluid in the middle ear; and tumors, such as cholesteatoma. Prior infections or perforations may have left scars on the tympanic membrane. A polyethylene ventilatory tube (grommet) placed in the tympanic membrane for chronic infection will be visible to the examiner.

Otoscopes are made to two basic designs. The open or operating otoscope is so constructed that the physician can insert instruments through it into the ear canal. When the closed, or pneumatic, otoscope is in position, its interior forms a closed space continuous with the ear canal. Pressure and suction alternately applied to this

impacted cerumen   otorrhea

TM (tympanic membrane)   myringitis

The tympanic membrane is slightly injected and deeply retracted.

SOM (serous otitis media)   aerotitis, barotitis

hemotympanum   cholesteatoma

Ramsay Hunt syndrome, zoster oticus

PE (poly; polyethylene tube)

space by means of a short rubber tube attached to a rubber bulb (or inserted in the physician's mouth) will move the tympanic membrane in and out unless the membrane is fixed by disease. This method is principally useful in children. The mobility of the tympanic membrane can also be tested by having the subject swallow while pinching the nostrils together or perform the Valsalva maneuver.

Both TM's move on Valsalva.

Hearing can be tested in various ways. Pure-tone audiometry with sophisticated electronic equipment in a soundproof booth is the method used by otologists, and may also be a part of school and industrial hearing testing, but it is not included in a standard physical examination. A rough notion of auditory acuity can be obtained by testing the examinee's ability to hear the spoken and whispered voice at various distances, with first one ear and then the other occluded. The subject's ability to hear a ticking watch held at various distances from the ear can also be compared with that of a person having normal hearing. Auditory discrimination can be tested by noting how well the subject can distinguish pairs of words differing in only one consonant, such as *back/bat* and *cool/pool*.

auditory threshold   audiogram   decibels

deafness, hearing impairment, hearing loss   threshold shift

presbycusis   discrimination, *scrim*

hyperacusis Willisii

Hearing loss can be of two types: conductive and neurosensory. Conductive hearing loss results from disease or injury of middle ear structures, neurosensory loss from malfunction of the acoustic nerve due to aging (presbycusis), noise exposure, or certain drugs and chemicals. Both conductive and neurosensory hearing loss can exist together in varying degrees. Two tests of value in distinguishing types of hearing impairment are the Rinne and the Weber test, both requiring the use of a tuning fork.

The Weber lateralizes to the right.

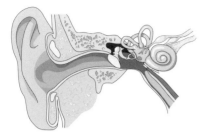

In the Rinne test, the examiner notes whether the subject can hear the sound of the vibrating fork better (that is, longer, as it gradually ceases to vibrate) by air conduction or by bone conduction. Air conduction is tested by placing the prongs of the vibrating fork near the external auditory meatus. Bone conduction is tested by placing the shank of the vibrating fork against the mastoid process (the bony prominence behind the external ear). With an intact acoustic nerve, the vibrations of the fork will still be audible by air conduction even when they can no longer be heard by bone conduction. When this is not the case, conductive hearing loss rather than neurosensory loss is likely. In the Weber test the examiner touches the shank of the vibrating fork to the middle of the subject's forehead. If the sound of the fork seems louder in the ear whose hearing is impaired, the impairment is conductive. If the sound of the fork seems fainter in the impaired ear, the impairment is neural.

air-bone gap

The assessment of **equilibrium** is usually performed by observing the patient's gait, particularly when walking a line (heel-to-toe walking), and testing the ability to stand erect with eyes closed without swaying or falling (Romberg test). The sensitivity of the Romberg test can be enhanced by having the subject stand with one foot in front of the other (tandem Romberg). Another test of vestibular function requires the patient to observe the location of some object (such as the examiner's forefinger), close the eyes, and touch the object. Past-pointing (failure to touch the object) suggests vestibular disease in a patient with normal coordination. The caloric test is occasionally used to assess vestibular function. Warmed or chilled water is gently injected with a syringe into the ear canal, one side being tested at a time. The sensation of vertigo and observable nystagmus indicate an intact vestibular apparatus on the side being tested. Persistence of this response for several minutes suggests abnormal sensitivity of the balance center to stimulation.

equilibrium, balance	Dix-Hallpike test	
caloric stimulation		
tandem gait, walking	Romberg, tandem Romberg	*past-pointing*

Exercises for Chapter 20

Review and Summarize

A. Multiple Choice

___ 1. The inner ear contains the following structures:
   a. Tympanic membrane and three small bones.
   b. Cochlea and vestibular apparatus.
   c. Pinna and auditory meatus.
   d. Auditory tube and eardrum.

___ 2. The caloric test is done with the use of
   a. Solid food.
   b. Alcohol.
   c. Water.
   d. Thermometer.

___ 3. The assessment of a person's ability to stand erect without falling or listing to one side is called
   a. Weber test.
   b. Past-pointing test.
   c. Heel-to-toe test.
   d. Romberg test.

___ 4. In older men there is a definite correlation between earlobe creases and
   a. Kidney disease.
   b. Liver disease.
   c. Heart disease.
   d. Inner ear disease.

B. Fill in the Blank

1. The pinna is composed of _____ tissue.

2. Two common tuning fork hearing tests are the _____ and _____.

3. Examination of the ear canal and tympanic membrane is performed with a(n) _____.

C. Short Answer

1. List the two types of hearing loss and their causes.

_____

_____

_____

_____

2. List the three main divisions of the ear.

_____   _____   _____

3. List abnormalities of the tympanic membrane that can be seen on examination.

_____

_____

_____

4. Write a short definition of the following terms. If you can, condense the definition into just a few words or a single synonym that you feel more comfortable with.

   a. Antihelix (or anthelix)_____

   b. Air-bone gap _____

   c. Cholesteatoma_____

   d. Valsalva maneuver_____

   e. Audiometry _____

   f. Tandem gait _____

   g. Gait _____

   h. Equilibrium _____

   i. Decibel_____

   j. Otorrhea_____

Pause and Reflect

Using different colored highlighters or crayons, underline or highlight important points or main ideas of the chapter. Circle key words. Use symbols meaningful to you (such as stars, asterisks, exclamation point, question mark, etc.) to mark key words and phrases. Summarize the information you thought most important from the chapter. If you had any questions, write those out to share with classmates or to ask your instructor.

_____

_____

_____

_____

_____

_____

Relate and Remember

Think of a metaphor that completes this statement: The human ear is like a _____.
Use a visual or a verbal metaphor. You may fill in the blank with the name of an object or draw (or cut out of a magazine) a picture representing one or more important points. Explain your choice.

_____

_____

_____

_____

_____

_____

Collaborate and Share

Stage a press conference with the parts of the ear. Assign students to represent the individual structures of the external, middle, and inner ear (pinna, external auditory canal, eardrum, tympanic membrane, and so on). Have these students hold signs indicating the part they represent. Remaining class members take turns asking questions of the parts about their function, symptoms of disease, etc. For example, "Pinna, I see you've undergone piercing. What kind of complications might you be at risk for?" or "My question is directed to all of the parts of the ear. How many of you are visible on external inspection?"

Explain and Learn

Working in pairs, take turns pointing out and explaining the important points or main idea of each paragraph or section in this chapter.

Relax and Play

1. With students divided into groups, each group selects a different game show ("Who Wants to be a Millionaire," "Jeopardy," "Hollywood Squares," etc.) and creates an "episode" using questions and answers related to this chapter. The games are presented using contestants from other groups. The class then votes on the best game presented.

2. Fold a blank piece of paper in half three times so that when unfolded there are eight squares. Write one thing you learned in each square. Move around the room, asking other students to define or explain an item on your sheet. That student then signs the square. The student who gets all eight squares signed first wins.

Generalize and Apply

Write a statement of something you learned from this chapter and how you think it will help you in your life or career. Crumple the sheet of paper into a "snowball." When the instructor says "go," toss the "snowball" into the air for other students to catch. When called on by the instructor, students then read the statements from the snowballs they caught to the rest of the class.

Compare and Contrast

What is the difference between the *eardrum* and the *tympanic membrane*? Are there any similarities? Why might confusion exist between these terms?

_____

_____

_____

_____

_____

_____

_____

_____

Extrapolate and Project

Auditory discrimination is important in the practice of medical transcription. There are many similar sounding terms whose meaning is not always ascertained from context. Identify terms in this chapter that might be difficult to distinguish in a dictated report. Discuss ways in which auditory discrimination skills might be refined.

_____

_____

_____

_____

_____

_____

_____

_____

_____

_____

_____

_____

21

Examination of the Nose, Throat, Mouth, and Teeth

Examination of the nose begins with external inspection for developmental abnormalities, traumatic deformities, enlargement (rhinophyma), nodules, ulcers, and other cutaneous lesions. The interior of each nostril is then viewed with a beam of light from a head mirror or other source. When a head mirror is used, the nostril is gently dilated with a bivalve nasal speculum. Alternatively, a cone-shaped speculum larger than those used for ear examination can be attached to an otoscope. The interior of the nose is inspected for septal deviation or perforation; mucosal edema, injection, ulcers, erosions, or polyps; discharge, hemorrhage, foreign bodies, and tumors. The sense of smell can be tested if necessary by having the subject try to identify familiar substances such as coffee or cinnamon by smell alone.

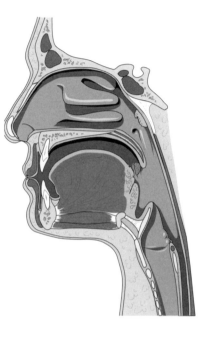

> Nose: Nasal passages are clear and no lesions are noted.
>
> ala nasi   columella   naris   septum   turbinate   middle meatus   vibrissae
>
> The nares are patent.
>
> depressed nasal bridge   saddle nose
>
> (acne) rosacea   rhinophyma
>
> *alar flaring*   transverse crease
>
> *allergic salute*   *rabbit nose*
>
> septal deviation, erosion, perforation   mucosa, mucous membrane
>
> K area (Kiesselbach area)
>
> rhinorrhea   inspissated mucus
>
> atrophic, hypertrophic, vasomotor rhinitis
>
> The middle and inferior turbinates are pale and boggy, with watery secretions.
>
> rhinitis medicamentosa   polyps   ozena

The **paranasal sinuses** are irregular cavities within certain bones of the skull. They are lined with mucous membrane and communicate with the nasal cavity by very small openings. They cannot be examined directly, but thickening of their lining membranes and accumulations of fluid due to infection can sometimes be detected by transillumination. If a small electric light is placed against appropriate parts of the head and face or inside the mouth in a darkened room, a deep ruddy glow can be seen through the skin. The examiner can judge from the intensity and configuration of this glow whether the sinus cavities are filled with air, as they should be, or with mucus or pus. (This method is far inferior to x-ray, CT scan, and MRI for diagnosis of sinus disease.)

Learning Objectives

After careful study of this chapter, you should be able to:

Discuss the methods of assessment and findings associated with examination of the nose.

Describe transillumination of the paranasal sinuses.

Identify terminology associated with the examination of the oral cavity.

Name the structures assessed on examination of the throat.

Define indirect laryngoscopy.

Name conditions that impart characteristic odors to the breath.

For Quick Reference

accumulation of fluid
acne rosacea
ala nasi
alar flaring
alcoholic breath
allergic salute
alveolar abscess
aphthae
aphthous ulcer
atrophic rhinitis
atrophy
bite line
bivalve nasal speculum
black hairy tongue
boggy turbinates
breath odor
buccal mucosa
canker sore
caries
caviar tongue
choanae
cobblestone tongue
columella
cone-shaped speculum
copious purulent postnasal discharge
crossbite
cutaneous lesion
cutaneous lesion of nose
debris in the tonsillar crypts
denture
depressed nasal bridge
dilatation of lingual papilla
dilated papillae
dysplasia of enamel
edema
edentulous and compensated
edentulous and uncompensated
enanthem
epiglottis
epulis
erythroplakia
ethmoid sinus
eustachian orifice
exudative tonsillopharyngitis
false teeth
fauces
faucial pillars
fetid breath
fetor oris
fissured tongue
Fordyce spots
foreign body
fossa of Rosenmueller
foul breath
frenulum
frontal sinus
fruity breath
furrowed tongue

---

ethmoid, frontal, maxillary, sphenoid sinus   paranasal sinuses

edema and tenderness over the left frontal sinus

The sinuses show no percussion tenderness, but he sounds like he is stuffy and has some nasal congestion.

Transillumination shows relative opacification of the left maxillary antrum, sinus.

For the examination of the **oral cavity**, the subject is instructed to open the mouth widely. The physician directs a beam of light into the mouth, gently using a tongue depressor to move lips or tongue as needed to improve the view. The buccal mucosa, the palate, and all surfaces of the tongue are inspected for petechiae, ulcers, tumors, leukoplakia, and signs of injury. The upper surface of the tongue is observed particularly for abnormal roughness or smoothness, furrowing, fissuring, or dilated papillae. When the tongue is protruded for inspection, any tremulousness or lateral deviation due to neurologic disease can be noted.

buccal mucosa, frenulum, lingual tonsil, lingual papillae

aphthae, aphthous ulcer, canker sore   leukoplakia, erythroplakia

enanthem, Koplik spots   *morsicatio buccarum, bite line*

Fordyce spots   stomatitis   sloughing

high arched palate   torus palatinus

macroglossia   glossitis

atrophy, dilatation of lingual papillae

tongue: *black hairy, caviar, cobblestone*, fissured, furrowed, furry, *geographic*, smooth, strawberry

median rhomboid glossitis   ranula

Stensen duct   Wharton duct

The tongue protrudes in the midline.

salivation   ptyalism, sialorrhea

The examiner observes the number, shape, and alignment of the **teeth** and any mottling, staining, caries, cavities, or restorations (fillings). Note is made of chipped, cracked, or missing teeth, as well as any dental appliances (bridges, plates, retainers, orthodontic braces) in use. Occlusion (bite) can be assessed by having the subject bring the teeth together while the lips are held apart with a tongue depressor. The gums are inspected for swelling, inflammation, ulceration, abnormal coloring, hypertrophy, or retraction.

Dental: The teeth are in good repair and the gums are healthy.

A few molars are missing.

edentulous and *compensated*   compensated edentulism

dysplasia, mottling, pitting, staining **of enamel**   caries

gingivae, gums   gingival atrophy, hypertrophy, recession

epulis   pyorrhea (alveolaris)

lead, mercury, metal line   alveolar abscess   pericoronitis

occlusion   crossbite, malocclusion, overbite, underbite

bridge, denture, false teeth, partial, plate

orthodontic braces   bite plate

Inspection of the **pharynx** is performed by having the subject say "ah," which raises the soft palate and otherwise dilates the oropharynx, while the examiner presses down gently on the back of the tongue with a tongue depressor. Adjustments in the position of the examiner's head and in the light source permit assessment of the soft palate and uvula, the root of the tongue, the faucial pillars, the tonsils if present, and the posterior wall of the oropharynx. Mucosal lesions, paralysis of the soft palate, edema, injection, exudate, and postnasal discharge or hemorrhage can thus be noted.

fauces   faucial pillars   tonsillar fossa   uvula

pharyngopalatine, glossopalatine arch   Waldeyer ring

The uvula rises in the midline on phonation.

hyperactive gag reflex   paralysis of the right side of the soft palate

pharyngeal edema   gelatinous edema of the uvula

hypertrophy of the tonsils   debris in the tonsillar crypts

petechiae of the soft palate   deeply injected, beefy red

peritonsillar abscess, retropharyngeal abscess   quinsy

exudative tonsillopharyngitis   dirty gray, lacy exudate

membrane, pseudomembrane   copious purulent postnasal discharge

lymphoid hyperplasia of the posterior pharyngeal wall

This part of the physical examination may be the most convenient opportunity for the examiner to note any abnormal odor of the patient's breath. Besides dental and oral disease, infection in any part of the respiratory tract can impart a foul odor to the breath. Certain metabolic disorders (ketosis, uremia, hepatic failure) can impart characteristic odors to the breath due to excretion of abnormal gases by the lungs. Alcohol and paraldehyde as well as certain foods and condiments can also be detected in the breath as they are excreted by the lungs.

breath: alcoholic, fetid, foul, fruity, ketotic, mousy, musty, putrid

fetor oris

Inspection of both the **nasopharynx** and the **larynx** can be performed with an angled mirror inserted through the mouth into the oropharynx. These examinations are not routine but may be indicated in certain circumstances and are easily performed if the patient can cooperate. Sometimes the pharynx and palate are sprayed with topical anesthetic to prevent gagging during the examination. Indirect laryngoscopy is performed with an angled mirror much like a dentist's mirror but with

For Quick Reference

furry tongue
gagging
gelatinous edema of uvula
geographic tongue
gingivae
gingival atrophy
glossitis
glossopalatine arch
gums
hemorrhage
high arched palate
hyperactive gag reflex
hypertrophic rhinitis
hypertrophy of tonsils
hypopharynx
indirect laryngoscopy
inspissated mucus
K (Kiesselbach) area
ketotic breath
Koplik spots
lacy exudate
larynx
leukoplakia
lingual papillae
lingual tonsil
lymphoid hyperplasia
macroglossia
malocclusion
maxillary sinus
median rhomboid glossitis
missing molars
morsicatio buccarum
mottling of enamel
mousy breath
mucosal lesion
mucous membrane
musty breath
naris (pl. nares)
nasal cavity
nasal passage
nasopharynx
nodule of nose
occlusion
oral cavity
oropharynx
overbite
ozena
palate
pale turbinates
paralysis of soft palate
paranasal sinuses
patent nares
pericoronitis
peritonsillar abscess
petechiae of soft palate
pharyngeal edema
pharyngeal wall
pharyngopalatine

For Quick Reference

a longer handle. Light is provided by a head mirror or other adjustable source. The examiner inserts the mirror into the posterior pharynx, being careful to avoid contact with the soft palate or pharyngeal walls, and views the vocal cords while the subject says "eeee" in a high-pitched voice. Tumors, paralysis, or inflammatory lesions of the cords can be seen. In addition, foreign bodies or tumors of other parts of the hypopharynx can be noted.

> epiglottis   piriform sinus   vocal cords   phonation
> Indirect laryngoscopy shows normal vocal cord motion and no lesions.
> Discrete, bilateral, symmetrical, hyperkeratotic nodules are seen on the cords.

A smaller mirror is used to examine the nasopharynx (posterior rhinoscopy). The technique is largely the same but the mirror is directed upward to enable the examiner to see the choanae, the adenoids if present, and the orifices of the eustachian tubes.

> posterior rhinoscopy   choanae
> eustachian orifice   torus tubarius
> fossa of Rosenmueller

Masses and other lesions in the mouth and pharynx can be palpated if necessary, the examiner donning a rubber glove and gently inserting one or two fingers to assess consistency or tenderness.

Exercises for Chapter 21

Review and Summarize

A. Multiple Choice

___ 1. The pharynx, palate, and nasopharynx are most often viewed during examination of the
   a. Ears.
   b. Nose.
   c. Throat.
   d. Sinuses.

___ 2. Glossitis is inflammation of the
   a. Uvula.
   b. Gums.
   c. Cheek.
   d. Tongue.

___ 3. The medical term for the upper jaw is
   a. Mastoid.
   b. Maxilla.
   c. Manubrium.
   d. Mandible.

B. Fill in the Blank

1. Indirect laryngoscopy is performed with an angled _____.

2. The _____ mucosa lines the inside of the cheek and mouth.

3. The paranasal sinuses are located within bones of the _____.

C. Short Answer

1. What does the physician look for during external examination of the nose?

_____

_____

_____

_____

2. Describe the technique of transillumination of the sinuses.

_____

_____

_____

_____

3. Other than food, drink, or medication, what medical conditions contribute to bad breath?

_____

_____

_____

_____

4. Write a short definition of the following terms. If you can, condense the definition into just a few words or a single synonym that you feel more comfortable with.

   a. Leukoplakia_____

   b. Papilla _____

   c. Sloughing _____

   d. Glossitis_____

   e. Fauces _____

   f. Exudate _____

   g. Purulent _____

   h. Choanae _____

Pause and Reflect

Type on a separate sheet or handwrite below an examination of the nose, throat, mouth, and teeth for a fictitious patient. Use as many terms as appropriate from the word list accompanying this chapter.

_____

_____

_____

_____

_____

_____

Relate and Remember

Create a visual representation of the examination of the nose, mouth, throat, and teeth. You may use a drawing, flow chart, graph, diagram, or metaphorical illustration. Explain, if necessary, how the visual representation relates to the exam.

Collaborate and Share

Label a blank sheet of paper with your name at the top and write a question requiring a short answer (less than a sentence) related to this chapter. Pass this paper to the student on your right, who will answer the question and then add a question of his or her own, as you answer the question on the paper received from the student on your left. Each sheet moves around the room until everyone has had a turn with every paper and you end up with the paper with your name at the top. Choose the best question(s) and answer(s) from your page to read aloud when called upon by your instructor.

Explain and Learn

Individually, using colored dots (or a drawn dot or star), mark what you feel is the most important point or line in each paragraph. If you feel there are multiple important points, rate them and mark the most important with, for example, a red dot, a secondary point with a yellow dot, and the least important point with a green dot. Once you have done this, share your findings with two or three classmates near you. Do you all agree? Discuss any differences of opinion and justify your final decisions.

Relax and Play

1. On a 3" x 5" card, each student writes a question pertaining to the chapter. The cards are collected by the instructor. The instructor, using a koosh ball, small stuffed animal, net bath sponge or some other soft object, asks the question, then tosses the object at random to an individual student who answers the question.

2. After reviewing the chapter as a class or in small groups, the instructor will announce "Go," and individual class members will "pop up" and call out one important fact learned, already known, or remembered about a topic or section in this chapter

Generalize and Apply

On a 3" x 5" card, write a statement of something you learned in this chapter and how you think this information will help you. Alternatively, write a question about something that has not yet been answered. Turn your card into your instructor as your "ticket" out of class.

Compare and Contrast

Compare and contrast the *paranasal sinuses*. What are the significant features of each? How are they similar in function and form? How do they differ?

_____

_____

_____

_____

_____

_____

_____

Extrapolate and Project

The author indicates that x-ray, CT scan, and MRI are superior to transillumination in the diagnosis of sinus disease. Speculate as to why a physician might choose to use transillumination in place of or prior to an x-ray or scan.

_____

_____

_____

_____

_____

_____

_____

_____

_____

_____

_____

_____

_____

_____

_____

22

Examination of the Thorax, Breasts, and Axillae

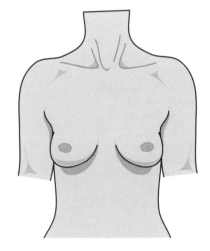

The thorax comprises roughly the upper half of the trunk, from the neck to the diaphragm, which at full inspiration lies just above the lower rib margins. Although in lay parlance the term *chest* refers only to the front of the thorax, the physician thinks of the chest as a three-dimensional anatomic region with a front, a back, and two sides. Some examiners proceed directly from the head and neck to the thorax, while others prefer to interpose examinations of the extremities or parts of the neurologic examination that can be performed before the patient undresses.

> The chest is symmetrical and respiratory excursions are full and equal.
> clavicle   scapula   scapular angle, spine
> sternum   manubrium   xiphoid
> midclavicular line   suprasternal notch, notch of Burns
> midscapular line   sternal angle, angle of Louis, Ludwig
> anterior, posterior axillary line   costal margins   intercostal spaces
> sternocostal, sternoclavicular joint   precordium

For the examination of the thorax the patient is undressed from the waist up and seated, if conscious and able to maintain that position. The physician observes the configuration of the chest walls, breathing movements, the skin, and the breasts before beginning the examination of the internal organs of the thorax. The examinations of the heart and the lungs are discussed in the next two chapters.

> Broadbent sign

The development and symmetry of the thorax are noted. Congenital deformities and injuries or diseases of the ribs or spine can alter the shape of the thorax. In pulmonary emphysema the anteroposterior diameter of the chest is often increased so that the rib cage approaches a cylindrical shape (barrel chest). Unless the subject is thin, the examiner will need to find some of the bony landmarks of the chest wall by palpation.

> increased AP (anteroposterior) diameter   barrel chest
> hyperinflation
> pectus carinatum, pigeon breast   funnel, hollow chest, pectus excavatum
> rachitic rosary   Harrison groove

Learning Objectives

After careful study of this chapter, you should be able to:

Distinguish between chest and thorax.

Discuss the development and symmetry of the thorax.

Identify terminology used to assess breathing movements.

Describe the examination of the breasts and axillae.

Name the areas of inspection on a breast exam.

For Quick Reference

Movements of the chest wall associated with breathing can be influenced by a number of factors, including, of course, the rate and rhythm of breathing itself. A patient with severe dyspnea may use muscles of the neck and upper chest to enhance lung filling that are not normally involved in breathing (accessory muscles of respiration). When inspiration is partly obstructed, it can cause retraction (sucking in) of the soft tissues between the ribs, above the clavicles, and in the epigastrium. When expiration is partly obstructed, it can cause bulging of soft tissues in the same areas. The symmetry of breathing movements can be affected by anything that reduces the depth of breathing on one side of the chest—atelectasis, paralysis, or severe pain on chest wall movement due to trauma such as rib fracture or disease such as pleurisy.

accessory muscles (of respiration)
intercostal and suprasternal bulging, retractions
guarding, splinting   costochondritis, Tietze syndrome

The physician inspects all surfaces of the chest for cutaneous lesions, surgical or traumatic scars, swellings, or masses, noting pigment and hair distribution (including axillary hair) and palpating abnormal areas to assess their consistency and note any tenderness. The **breasts** are palpated in both sexes, but in women the procedure is more elaborate. The female breasts are inspected for abnormalities of shape, lack of symmetry, deformity or retraction of nipples, cutaneous changes, surgical scars, and lack of mobility when the arms are raised over the head. They are systematically palpated for masses or tenderness in both the erect and supine postures. Finally the axillae are palpated to detect enlarged or tender lymph nodes or other lesions.

scanty axillary hair
The breasts are pendulous and generally lumpy, without tenderness or dominant lump.
areola   glands of Montgomery
retracted nipple   supernumerary nipple, polythelia
axillary tail of Spence   upper outer quadrant
Paget disease of the nipple   fissuring of the nipple
pigmented areolae   gynecomastia
peau d'orange   dominant lump
nipple bleeding, discharge   milk, colostrum
quadrantic massage
hidradenitis suppurativa   axillary lymphadenopathy

Exercise for Chapter 22

Review and Summarize

A. Multiple Choice

___ 1. Retraction of the chest wall on inspiration can be caused by
    a. Partial obstruction of the airway.
    b. Overexpansion of the lungs.
    c. Symmetry of breathing motions.
    d. Failure of accessory muscles of respiration.
    e. All of the above.

___ 2. Which one of the following findings would be of specific concern on breast examination?
    a. Oval-shaped breasts.
    b. Nipple retraction.
    c. Pendulous breasts.
    d. Eversion of nipples.
    e. Both A and D.

B. Fill in the Blank

1. Patients with the respiratory disease _____ often have an increased chest diameter, giving the chest a barrel shape.

2. The thorax spans the upper half of the body from the _____ to the _____.

C. Short Answer

1. The examiner can discern several important findings just by looking at the patient's thorax. List those things that can be noted with visual inspection only.

_____

_____

_____

_____

_____

_____

_____

2. Write a short definition of the following terms. If you can, condense the definition into just a few words or a single synonym that you feel more comfortable with.

a. Xiphoid _____

b. Clavicle _____

c. Costal _____

d. Rachitic _____

e. Accessory _____

f. Guarding _____

g. Splinting _____

h. Supernumerary _____

i. Quadrant _____

j. Axillae _____

k. Pendulous _____

Pause and Reflect

Read this chapter aloud, by yourself or taking turns with other students. If you don't know the meaning or pronunciation of a word, look it up. As you read, pause and reflect on key points at the end of each section. Make notes in the margins of your book, mark with dots or stars, and draw lines from key ideas to subordinate points. Summarize your reading in outline form below.

_____

_____

_____

_____

_____

_____

_____

Relate and Remember

Using this outline of the thorax, list 3 to 5 terms for each area that the physician might use to describe the findings in that area.

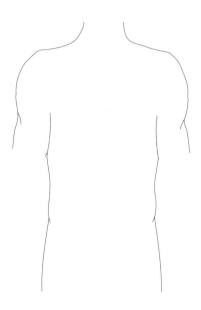

Collaborate and Share

On a 3" x 5" card, write a question pertaining to the chapter. The instructor will collect the cards and divide the class into small groups. Each group gets a portion of the questions to answer and share with the class.

Explain and Learn

List everything you know about this chapter. As a group, pick 1 to 3 most important points and share with the class.

_____

_____

_____

_____

_____

_____

Relax and Play

With all members of the class standing, choose a term pertaining to the thorax, breasts, or axillae that begins with the letter A and make a statement beginning with this term, such as "Axillary hair may be scanty." The next student makes a statement beginning with the letter B, such as "Breasts are examined for abnormalities." Continue through the alphabet, with each student taking the next letter. Anyone who cannot come up with a statement sits down. The winner is the last person standing.

Generalize and Apply

Write a letter to a friend or family member explaining one thing you have learned in this chapter and how you will use that knowledge in your work.

_____

_____

_____

_____

_____

_____

_____

_____

_____

_____

_____

_____

_____

_____

Compare and Contrast

What is the difference between the terms *thorax* and *chest* as used by a patient and by a physician?

_____

_____

_____

_____

Extrapolate and Project

Examine literature on breast self-examination. Who should do breast self-examination and why? How often should it be performed? What is the current thinking on the relationship between breast self-examination and early cancer detection? How does early cancer detection influence life expectancy?

_____

_____

_____

_____

_____

_____

_____

_____

_____

_____

_____

_____

_____

23

Examination of the Heart

Books much larger than this one have been devoted exclusively to the performance and interpretation of procedures for the assessment of cardiovascular function and the detection of cardiovascular disease. Even a routine physical examination may include many of these procedures, and when cardiac disease is suspected or recognized, many more will be used. Because the circulatory system extends throughout the entire body, tests of its integrity and function are included in the examination of various regions, and so may be found recorded in various parts of the physical examination report. For example, inspection of the retinal vasculature is performed as part of the eye examination, and so recorded. Peripheral pulses are felt as the neck, arms, and legs are being examined, and so on.

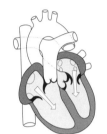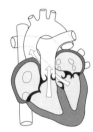

Heart: Regular without murmurs, gallops, or rubs.

Very little information can be obtained about the structure of the heart through direct examination. Virtually the entire cardiac examination consists of observation of the function of the heart—the rate, regularity, and intensity of ventricular contractions, the resulting impulses imparted to the circulating blood and to the chest wall, and the sounds generated by cardiac contraction and the movement of blood. Congenital anomalies, valvular disease, arrhythmias, pericardial effusions and adhesions, ventricular dilatation and hypertrophy, congestive heart failure—all must be detected or inferred by examination of cardiac function. X-rays, cardiograms, and other noninvasive and invasive diagnostic procedures can yield more precise data about structural alterations in the heart and great vessels, but even these depend largely on assessment of cardiac function.

Examined in recumbent, left lateral, sitting, and standing positions, as well as bending forward and squatting.

precordium

Examination of the heart is ideally carried out with the patient seated and undressed from the waist up. Hence it logically follows the examination of the thorax, breasts, and axillae. The examiner has already noted such findings as pallor, flushing, cyanosis, respiratory distress, and dilated jugular veins. The anterior chest wall is inspected for pulsations and the point at which the cardiac impulse is strongest (point of maximal intensity, PMI) is found by palpation. The examiner's fingers not only locate this point but also detect any abnormalities associated

Learning Objectives

After careful study of this chapter, you should be able to:

List the functions of the heart that can be assessed by observation.

Explain why findings in other body systems relate to assessment of the heart.

Explain the process of palpation and the findings relevant to it.

Name findings obtainable on cardiac auscultation.

Define normal and abnormal heart sounds, giving examples of each.

Discuss the detection of murmurs and their role in assessing valvular anatomy.

Describe other tests of cardiac function that can be performed.

Identify terminology related to the anatomy of the heart.

For Quick Reference

with the heartbeat, such as a heaving of the chest wall due to unduly intense cardiac contractions, thrills due to passage of blood through abnormally narrowed valves or other orifices, and shocks from abnormally abrupt closure of valves in hypertension. Percussion can also be used to assess cardiac size and shape, although many examiners doubt the validity of this procedure. (Percussion is described in the next chapter.)

> The PMI is in the left fifth interspace at the midclavicular line.
>
> The PMI is palpated 13 cm to the left of the midsternal line.
>
> A precordial thrill is palpable.
>
> left parasternal lift, heave, shock
>
> Precordial palpation reveals a systolic thrill in the upper sternal area.
>
> Palpation of the precordium reveals a sustained ventricular apex beat and an atrial filling impulse.
>
> The left border of cardiac dullness is at the midclavicular line.

Auscultation provides more information about the heart than any other procedure. Stethoscopes used for cardiac auscultation have two chest pieces: a narrow, cone-shaped "bell" for lower pitched sounds and a wide, flat diaphragm for higher pitched sounds. The examiner changes back and forth from one to the other as needed during the examination. The stethoscope is applied to the chest in specific areas according to a basic routine, which may be varied as circumstances dictate. Four areas of the anterior chest are designated according to the valves whose sounds are best heard there: the mitral area, the pulmonic area, the aortic area, and the tricuspid area. The subject may need to change position, such as by leaning forward or lying on the left side, to enable the examiner to evaluate heart sounds adequately.

> dextrocardia   situs inversus

On auscultation the examiner hears regularly recurring sounds produced by the rhythmic contraction of the ventricles and associated phenomena. From these the rate, regularity, and intensity of ventricular contractions can be judged. In addition, the examiner listens for abnormal sounds: *murmurs*, caused by abnormal flow of blood through a valve or other orifice; *clicks* or *snaps*, caused by abnormal valve function; *rubs*, creaking or grating sounds caused by friction between the beating heart and an inflamed pericardium; *bruits*, caused by passage of blood through a narrowed artery; and others.

> **(pericardial) friction rub:** coarse, creaking, faint, grating, harsh, loud, scratchy, shuffling, soft
>
> pericardial knock

The normally beating heart produces two **sounds** in alternation, traditionally represented as *lub-dup*. The first heart sound, or S1, which is louder, deeper in pitch, and longer, results from contraction of the ventricles and closure of the mitral and tricuspid valves. For practical purposes it is considered synchronous with the beginning of systole (the stage of ventricular contraction, which sends blood through the aorta and pulmonary artery). The second heart sound, S2, results from closure of the aortic and pulmonic valves just after systole ends. S2 is taken as the beginning of diastole (the stage of ventricular relaxation and refilling). The first and second heart sounds heard at specific valve areas are sometimes so designated: A1, the first heart sound at the aortic valve area; P2, the second heart sound heard at the pulmonic valve area; and so on.

> A2 is equal to P2.
>
> Heart tones are distant, muffled, reduced, weak.
>
> accentuated, increased M1

The absolute and relative intensities of S1 and S2 vary from place to place on the chest and may even vary from beat to beat. Either sound can be abnormally accentuated or diminished and either can be reduplicated or split, that is, can consist of two not quite simultaneous components. Splitting of the second sound is often physiologic (normal), in which case it typically disappears during expiration. Two other heart sounds can occasionally be heard in a normal person: S3, due to ventricular filling in early diastole, and S4, due to atrial contraction in late diastole. Accentuation of either or both by disease can alter the regularly recurring *lub-dup* to a more complex sequence of sounds called a gallop. Accentuation of S3 produces what is called a ventricular gallop (something like *lub-dup-uh*), and accentuation of S4 produces an atrial gallop (something like *uh-lub-dup*).

> fixed, paradoxical, physiologic splitting of S2
>
> embryocardia, ticktock rhythm   atrial, ventricular gallop

Although an electrocardiogram is needed for precise diagnosis of **arrhythmias** (abnormalities in cardiac rhythm), auscultation can yield much valuable information about the rhythm. A slight or even marked variation in heart rate with the breathing cycle (increase on inspiration, decrease on expiration) is normal and is known as sinus arrhythmia. Occasional extra beats (extrasystoles, premature ventricular contractions) are also normal. Occurrence of a premature beat after each normal beat (coupling or bigeminy) is more ominous. Irregularities of the pulse are designated, somewhat whimsically, as regular irregularities (having a pattern, albeit abnormal) and irregular irregularities (wholly random, without discernible pattern). The examiner can obtain additional information about arrhythmias by correlating auscultatory findings with peripheral pulses. Cautious massage of one carotid sinus (located on either side of the neck near the origins of the internal carotid arteries) normally results in slowing of the pulse and can convert some arrhythmias to normal sinus rhythm.

Cardiac murmurs are produced by turbulence in the flow of blood passing forward through a stenotic valve, leaking back through an incompetent valve, or crossing from a place of higher to a place of lower pressure through an abnormal

For Quick Reference

rub
rumbling murmur
S1
S2
S3
S4
scratchy friction rub
seagull murmur
shuffling friction rub
sinus arrhythmia
sinus bradycardia
sinus tachycardia
situs inversus
soft friction rub
stenosis
stenotic valve
stethoscope
synchronous
systolic murmur
systolic thrill
tachyarrhythmia
tachycardia
ticktock rhythm
tilt test
to-and-fro murmur
tricuspid valve area
valvular click
valvular disease
valvular snap
venous hum
ventricular apex beat
ventricular contraction
ventricular dilatation
ventricular gallop
ventricular hypertrophy
ventricular refilling
ventricular relaxation
water-hammer pulse
weak heart tones

RSR (regular sinus rhythm)

sinus arrhythmia, bradycardia, tachycardia   *pulse deficit*

bigeminy, coupling   compensatory pause

pulsus alternans

bradyarrhythmia, tachyarrhythmia   carotid sinus massage

idioventricular rhythm

orifice, such as an interventricular septal defect. The diagnostician characterizes a murmur by recording its location (the point on the chest wall where it is heard best); its radiation or transmission (for example, to the carotid arteries or left axilla); its character, intensity (graded on a scale of 1 to 6; less often, 1 to 4), and duration; and its timing within the cardiac cycle. Valvular clicks and snaps are similarly characterized.

precordium   apex   base

On auscultation there is a short, high-pitched murmur best heard along the left sternal border.

A grade 2 blowing holosystolic murmur best heard along the left sternal border and disappearing after exercise.

Auscultation reveals a systolic murmur with a crescendo-decrescendo configuration beginning after S1, loudest in the right second intercostal space parasternally, which radiates to the neck, left sternal border, and apex.

best heard in the left lateral decubitus position

transmitted to the apex, axilla, base, carotids, neck

murmur: blowing, coarse, cooing-dove, crescendo, decrescendo, *diamond-shaped*, diminuendo, harsh, high-pitched, low-pitched, musical, rasping, rumbling, seagull

A murmur heard between S1 and S2 is called systolic, and a murmur heard between S2 and the succeeding S1 is called diastolic. Some systolic murmurs are of no consequence (functional or innocent murmurs). A holosystolic or pansystolic murmur lasts all the way from S1 to S2; a shorter murmur may be designated early, mid, or late systolic. A murmur can become more or less noticeable after physical exertion or on inspiration, expiration, or change of position (lying on the left side, squatting). A murmur can start soft and grow louder (crescendo), start loud and grow softer (decrescendo), or become first louder and then softer (crescendo-decrescendo or diamond-shaped murmur). Some murmurs not associated with valvular lesions are heard with little or no change throughout both systole and diastole (to-and-fro, machinery murmurs). By considering all the features of a murmur, the diagnostician can generally judge which valve, if any, is the source of the murmur, and whether it results from abnormal narrowing or tightness (stenosis) of a valve or backflow (regurgitation) of blood through an incompetent one.

Certain other tests of cardiac function and circulation are performed as indicated. In a tilt test, the pulse is counted with the subject in a recumbent position and again immediately after assumption of a sitting position. A significant rise in pulse

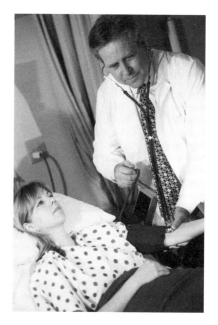

murmur: diastolic, presystolic, protodiastolic, systolic

(proto)diastolic rumble   aortic, pulmonic ejection click

a loud midsystolic click and a late systolic murmur

Graham Steell murmur   Austin Flint murmur

mitral opening snap   venous hum

or drop in blood pressure suggests hypovolemia and impending shock. **Pulsus paradoxus** is an exaggerated drop in systolic blood pressure on inspiration, caused by constrictive pericarditis or pericardial tamponade due to effusion or hemorrhage. The physician tests for pulsus paradoxus by having the subject inspire deeply and noting any weakening in peripheral pulses. In doubtful cases a sphygmomanometer can be used to demonstrate a drop in arterial pressure.

Tilt test is negative.

paradoxical pulse, pulsus paradoxus

cardiac, pericardial tamponade

Pulse pressure is the arithmetical difference between systolic and diastolic pressures. Hence if the patient's blood pressure is 148/68, the pulse pressure is 80. A "wide" pulse pressure can result from various causes, including hypovolemia, vasodilatation, and aortic regurgitation. It may be manifested as a visible jerking of the head or extremities synchronous with heartbeat. On palpation, the peripheral pulses have a particularly thumping or bounding character, the so-called Corrigan or water-hammer pulse. Capillary pulsations (Quincke pulse) may be evident in the nail beds and elsewhere as a rhythmic blushing synchronous with heartbeat.

bishop's nod   Musset sign

Corrigan, water-hammer pulse   pistol shot pulse

Quincke pulse, capillary pulsations

Exercises for Chapter 23

Review and Summarize

A. Multiple Choice

___ 1. Which technique provides more information about the heart than any other?
a. Auscultation.
b. Percussion.
c. Chest x-ray.
d. Electrocardiogram (EKG).

___ 2. A sound caused by the abnormal flow of blood through a valve or other orifice is known as a
a. Murmur.
b. Thrill.
c. Gallop.
d. Snap.

___ 3. A slight or marked variation in heart rate with the breathing cycle is known as
a. Tachycardia.
b. Bradycardia.
c. Extrasystole.
d. Sinus arrhythmia.

___ 4. Heart murmurs are most often graded on a scale of
a. 1 to 2.
b. 1 to 4.
c. 1 to 6.
d. 1 to 10.

B. Fill in the Blank

1. The first heart sound is also known as _____.

2. _____ is the stage of ventricular contraction that sends blood through the aorta and pulmonary artery.

3. Massage of the _____ sinus can slow the pulse and sometimes convert abnormal rhythm to normal rhythm.

4. The _____ are traditionally represented as "lub-dup."

C. Short Answer

1. The four areas of the anterior chest are designated according to which valves?

_____

_____

_____

_____

2. What is the difference between a *crescendo murmur*, a *decrescendo murmur*, and a *crescendo-decrescendo murmur*?

_____

_____

_____

_____

3. Write a short definition of the following terms. If you can, condense the definition into just a few words or a single synonym that you feel more comfortable with.

   a. Click _____

   b. Rub _____

   c. Apex _____

   d. Paradoxical _____

   e. Bigeminy_____

   f. Idioventricular _____

   g. Precordium_____

   h. Crescendo _____

   i. Gallop _____

Pause and Reflect

Type on a separate sheet or handwrite below the physical examination of the heart for a fictitious patient, using the criteria described in this chapter. Use as many terms as appropriate from the word list in the chapter. Be sure to indicate pertinent negatives as well as positive findings.

_____

_____

_____

_____

_____

_____

_____

_____

Relate and Remember

Take a sheet of paper and draw lines to create four columns, labeled A through D. List five important things to remember about the chapter. Put these in column A. In column B, next to each of the items to remember, write the name of an object that might help you to remember the fact. In column C, write the name of a place that might help you to remember the fact. In column D, write a description of a visual image with which you can associate the fact in column A.

Collaborate and Share

After you have read the chapter, form groups of 3 to 5. Divide the chapter so that each group has a portion. Re-read your section. As a group, write questions based on your section. They may be multiple choice, short answer, or fill in the blank. The number of questions will depend on how large a section of the chapter your group is covering. Pass your questions to the next group, working clockwise around the room, until every group has had the opportunity to answer all the questions.

Explain and Learn

In groups of 3 to 5 students, with each group assigned a different section of the chapter, discuss and agree on the important points or main ideas. Put them into your own words. Select one person to present your summary to the class.

Relax and Play

1. With students divided into groups, each group selects a different game show ("Who Wants to be a Millionaire," "Jeopardy," "Hollywood Squares," etc.) and creates an "episode" using questions and answers related to this chapter. The games are presented using contestants from other groups. The class then votes on the best game presented.

2. Fold a blank piece of paper in half three times so that when unfolded there are eight squares. Write one thing you learned in each square. Move around the room, asking other students to define or explain an item on your sheet. That student then signs the square. The student who gets all eight squares signed first wins.

Generalize and Apply

Tests of the integrity and function of the cardiovascular system are reported in various parts of the physical examination report. Obtain a dozen or more sample H&P reports and circle every reference to the cardiovascular system made outside of the actual heart exam. Summarize these references below.

_____

_____

_____

_____

_____

_____

_____

Compare and Contrast

Compare and contrast these abnormal heart sounds: _murmurs, clicks_ or _snaps, rubs,_ and _bruits_. How do they differ from each other in origin and in sound? How are they similar?

_____

_____

_____

_____

_____

Extrapolate and Project

Although new medical and surgical treatments have reduced the number of deaths attributed to it, heart disease remains the leading cause of death in the U.S. There are risk factors outside of a patient's control—age, family history, and personal history of heart disease—but there are other risk factors within a patient's control. Identify these risk factors and discuss how patients can work in partnership with their physicians to reduce the incidence of heart disease. Use your other textbooks and outside resources as necessary.

_____

_____

_____

_____

_____

_____

_____

_____

_____

_____

_____

_____

_____

_____

_____

_____

_____

_____

_____

_____

24

Examination of the Lungs

Physical assessment of the lungs naturally follows examination of the heart. The subject is seated if possible and undressed from the waist up. The examiner has already noted any asymmetry or other deformity of the thorax and any signs of respiratory distress.

> The lungs are clear to auscultation and percussion.

Evaluation of the lungs is performed almost entirely by the techniques of auscultation and percussion (A&P). The passage of air into and out of the lungs during normal respiration produces a characteristic sequence of sounds, as heard through the chest wall with a stethoscope. Structural changes in the breathing apparatus due to disease or injury cause predictable changes in the quality and loudness of the breath sounds and can induce abnormal sounds as well. The subject is instructed to breathe somewhat more deeply than normal with the mouth open (so as to avoid extraneous sounds caused by the passage of air through the nose) while the examiner listens at specific places on the front and back of the chest. Ordinarily the diaphragm chest piece of the stethoscope is preferred for this purpose.

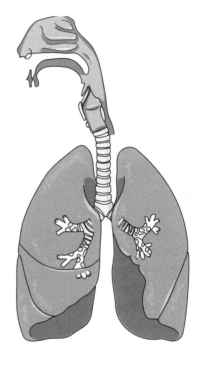

> lung fields   apex, apical area   base, basilar area
> lower, upper lobe

Normal inspiration and expiration yield a faint sighing or whispering sound called vesicular breathing. This sound might be compared to that of a steady, gentle breeze passing through and stirring the leaves of a tree. The inspiratory phase of vesicular breathing is slightly longer than the expiratory phase, and slightly louder. In fact, the expiratory phase may be inaudible. When the two phases of respiration are about equal in intensity, one speaks of bronchovesicular breathing. When the expiratory phase is louder, the term bronchial (or tubular) breathing is applied.

> **breathing (breath sounds)**: amphoric, bronchial, bronchovesicular, cavernous, cogwheel, tubular, vesicular

Certain abnormal conditions can superimpose **abnormal sounds** (rhonchi, rales, or rubs) on the basic inspiratory-expiratory breath sounds. A *rhonchus* is a

Learning Objectives

After careful study of this chapter, you should be able to:

Explain the method by which the lungs are examined.

Differentiate between inspiratory and expiratory breath sounds.

Define *rhonchi*, *rales*, and *rubs*.

Describe maneuvers that elicit abnormal breath sounds.

Name conditions related to the absence of breath sounds.

Identify terminology related to examination of the lungs.

Explain percussion and its role as a diagnostic maneuver.

For Quick Reference

continuous sound such as is made by a whistle or horn. Rhonchi result from passage of air through a respiratory passage narrowed by bronchospasm (in asthma), swelling, thickened secretions, or tumor. Rhonchi vary widely in pitch and intensity. In asthma, rhonchi of many different pitches may be heard together ("musical chest"). A *rale* is an irregular, discontinuous sound, like bubbling fluid, crackling paper, or popping corn. Rales are due to passage of air through fluid—mucus, pus, edema fluid, or blood—or to the sudden expansion of small air passages that have been plugged or sealed by mucus. Asking a subject with rales or rhonchi to cough and then listening again to the breath sounds may supply helpful information about the character or severity of the underlying disorder. The examiner carefully notes in what part of the chest and at what part of the breathing cycle rhonchi or rales are heard or are loudest.

---

adventitious breath sounds

rhonchi: coarse, high-pitched, humming, low-pitched, musical, *post-tussive*, sibilant, sonorous, whistling

rales: bibasilar, bubbling, coarse, crackling crepitant, moist, *post-tussive*, sticky

Inspiratory rhonchi are heard over the right upper chest.

There are fine crepitant rales at both bases.

Expiration is accompanied by wheezing audible without a stethoscope.

A pleural friction rub is a creaking, grating, or rubbing sound caused by friction between inflamed pleural surfaces during breathing. Sometimes it resembles the sound of a creaking shoe, sometimes the sound of two tree branches rubbing together in the wind. It may be faint or conspicuous, prolonged or brief (that is, occurring at just one point in the respiratory cycle). When both air and fluid are present in the pleural cavity (hydropneumothorax), a bubbling or splashing sound can sometimes be heard with the stethoscope if the subject is shaken; this is known as a succussion splash.

(pleural) friction rub: coarse, creaking, faint, grating, harsh, loud, scratchy, shuffling, soft

Hamman sign   succussion splash

distant, faint, muffled, reduced breath sounds

egophony   pectoriloquy

bronchophony   whispered pectoriloquy   D'Espine sign

Reduction or absence of breath sounds over a part of the chest wall can result from any of several conditions—collapse of lung tissue (atelectasis), consolidation of lung tissue due to pneumonia, presence in the pleural space of air (pneumothorax), blood (hemothorax), pus (empyema), or fluid (hydrothorax, pleural effusion), and tumor. Some of these can be differentiated by determining how well the sound of the subject's voice passes through the involved area. When the subject says "ee," the examiner hears "ee" through normal lung, "ay" through consolidated lung or air in the pleural space. Enhancement of sound transmission by consolidated lung is called bronchophony. Whispered pectoriloquy means that even whispered words are clearly heard through the stethoscope.

In another test using the subject's voice, the examiner places the flat of the hand over various parts of the chest while the subject repeatedly says "bananas," "ninety-nine," or some other word or phrase yielding similar resonance and overtones. The vibration felt by the examiner, known as vocal fremitus, is enhanced by consolidation of lung, damped by intervening air or fluid.

tactile, vocal fremitus	Ewart sign

Percussion of the chest, though a valuable diagnostic procedure, has been largely supplanted by x-rays. This procedure is based on the fact that structural alterations within the thorax change the behavior of sound waves that are produced when the chest wall is tapped. In the standard technique, called mediate percussion, the examiner places the palm of one hand with outspread fingers against the subject's chest and taps the back of the middle finger smartly with the flexed tip of the other middle finger. The percussion note over normal lung tissue is described as resonant. In atelectasis, consolidation, or pleural effusion the note is dull or even flat; in pneumothorax or emphysema it may be hyperresonant or even tympanitic (drumlike). Percussion can be used to find the levels of the right and left hemidiaphragms in inspiration and expiration and to trace the left border of an enlarged heart.

percussion

percussion note: dull, flat, hyperresonant, resonant, tympanitic

atelectasis   pneumothorax   hydrothorax

As a rough test for obstructive pulmonary disease, the examiner may instruct the patient to blow out a match held several inches from the mouth without pursing the lips.

Fails match test at 3 inches.

Exercises for Chapter 24

Review and Summarize

A. Multiple Choice

___ 1. When the sound heard during the expiratory phase of breathing is louder than during the inspiratory phase, this is termed
    a. Bronchovesicular breathing.
    b. Vesicular breathing.
    c. Bronchial breathing.
    d. Adventitious breathing.

___ 2. A pleural friction rub sounds like
    a. Bubbling.
    b. Crackling.
    c. Grating.
    d. Honking.

___ 3. The percussion note over normal lung tissue is described as
    a. Resonant.
    b. Musical.
    c. Tympanitic.
    d. Flat.

B. Fill in the Blank

1. The faint sigh or whispering noise heard on normal breathing is known as _____ breath sounds.

2. The vibration felt by the examiner's hand over the patient's chest with the patient speaking is called

_____.

C. Short Answer

1. Why is the patient instructed to breathe through the mouth on examination of the lungs?

_____

_____

_____

2. List the conditions that could cause a reduction or absence of breath sounds.

_____

_____

_____

_____

_____

3. Write a short definition of the following terms. If you can, condense the definition into just a few words or a single synonym that you feel more comfortable with.

a. Adventitious _____

b. Crepitant _____

c. Pectoriloquy _____

d. Succussion _____

e. Egophony _____

f. Bronchophony _____

g. Fremitus _____

h. Atelectasis _____

i. Hydrothorax _____

Pause and Reflect

Using different colored highlighters or crayons, underline or highlight important points or main ideas of the chapter. Circle key words. Use symbols meaningful to you (such as stars, asterisks, exclamation point, question mark, etc.) to mark key words and phrases. Summarize the information you thought most important from the chapter. If you had any questions, write those out to share with classmates or to ask your instructor.

_____

_____

_____

_____

_____

_____

_____

_____

Relate and Remember

Make a mind map for the lung exam using the conditions that can affect the lungs as the outer ring of circles. In the next ring of circles, list the examination findings that point to each condition.

Collaborate and Share

On a paper bag, write your name and the statement, "I want to know more about . . ." Pass the bag around the room. The other students write what they know about the question on a piece of paper and initial their answers, placing the paper inside the bag. When the bag returns to you, summarize the information in the bag and share the summary with the class.

Explain and Learn

Working in pairs, take turns pointing out and explaining the important points or main idea of each paragraph or section in this chapter.

Relax and Play

1. Using the words from #2 of the Short Answer questions or at least 10 terms from the word list in the chapter, write a poem or song that incorporates these terms in such a way as to reveal their meaning or use. If writing a song, you can use a familiar tune or rap style.

2. Working in groups of three, pantomime the physical examination of the lungs in a patient with emphysema. One student will be the patient, one the examining physician, and the other will narrate the examination process, describing the techniques and findings as the examination progresses. Switch roles and choose another lung condition, such as bronchitis, pneumothorax, and so on.

Generalize and Apply

The abbreviation *AP* can be used in a lung examination to mean "anterior and posterior" as well as "auscultation and percussion." Discuss the risk of abbreviation misuse in medical reports.

_____

_____

_____

_____

_____

_____

_____

_____

Compare and Contrast

1. What is the audible difference between *rhonchi* and *rales*?

    _____

    _____

    _____

2. What is the difference between the terms *atelectasis* and *pneumothorax*? How are they similar?

    _____

    _____

    _____

Extrapolate and Project

Based on your understanding of the lung examination from this chapter, what challenges might be faced by a medical transcriptionist in recording the results of this examination?

_____

_____

_____

_____

_____

_____

_____

_____

_____

_____

25

Examination of the Abdomen, Groins, Rectum, Anus, and Genitalia

The abdomen and pelvis comprise the lower half of the trunk, from the diaphragm to the perineum. Whereas the physician examines the thorax from all sides with the patient upright, the abdomen is approached almost exclusively from the ventral surface, and most of the examination is carried out with the patient supine. This is largely because the massive lumbar vertebrae, the pelvic bones, and their associated musculature preclude palpation, percussion, and auscultation of abdominal and pelvic organs from behind.

> The abdomen is soft and nontender, without palpable masses or enlarged organs.
>
> The abdomen is slightly distended and there is mild tenderness to deep palpation of the left lower quadrant. No rebound or guarding. No masses or organomegaly.

The patient lies supine (face up) in as comfortable a position as possible with arms relaxed at the sides. The abdomen is exposed from the costal margins to the pubes. A right-handed physician stands at the patient's right to facilitate palpation. As always when a new body region is exposed to view, the skin is first observed for any abnormal pigmentation, stretch marks (striae), surgical or traumatic scars, dilated veins, rashes, nodules, or other lesions. The umbilicus is inspected for signs of herniation or infection. The overall contour and symmetry of the abdomen are noted as well as any masses, pulsations, or visible peristalsis.

LLQ (left lower quadrant)

region: epigastric, hypogastric, periumbilical, suprapubic

LUQ (left upper quadrant)   navel, umbilicus

RLQ (right lower quadrant)   linea alba, linea nigra

RUQ (right upper quadrant)   stretch marks, striae

Cullen sign   (Grey) Turner sign

caput medusae   varices   colostomy, ileostomy   stoma

everted umbilicus   umbilical hernia   Sister Joseph sign

abdomen: distended, flat, obese, protuberant, scaphoid

diastasis recti   abdominal retraction on inspiration

apron   panniculus adiposus

incisional hernia, spigelian hernia

appendectomy scar   right, left paramedian scar

cholecystectomy incision   Pfannenstiel incision   hockey-stick incision

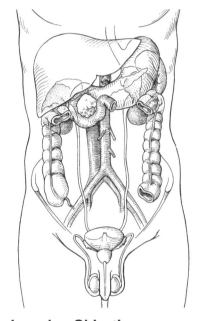

Learning Objectives

After careful study of this chapter, you should be able to:

Describe the abdominal and pelvic cavity and their contents.

List findings detectable on visual inspection of the abdomen and pelvis.

Describe the techniques of palpation, percussion, auscultation, and ballottement.

Classify types of tenderness by method of detection and associated conditions.

Distinguish among the various types of hernias.

Name the structures assessed on rectal exam for males and females.

Identify methods, equipment, structures and conditions related to the female pelvic exam.

For Quick Reference

abdominal retraction on inspiration
absent bowel sounds
acute abdomen
adnexa
anal canal
anal procidentia
anal prolapse
anal protrusion
anal verge
anoderm
anorchia
anteflexion
anteversion
anus
appendectomy scar
apron
ascites
balanitis
balanoposthitis
Ballance sign
ballotable
ballottement
Bartholin gland
bartholinitis
bimanual pelvic examination
bivalve speculum
Blumer rectal shelf
boardlike rigidity
boggy prostate
bowel sounds
BPH (benign prostatic hyperplasia)
Braxton-Hicks contractions
breech presentation
brown discharge
bruits of the renal arteries
bubo adenopathy
BUS (Bartholin glands, urethra, and
    Skene glands)
canal of Nuck
caput medusae
cephalic presentation
cervix
Chadwick sign
chancre
chandelier sign
cholecystectomy incision
circular sulci
circumcised
cockscomb deformity
colostomy
condyloma acuminatum
contour and symmetry of abdomen
costal margin
costovertebral angle tenderness
crabs
cryptorchism
cul-de-sac
Cullen sign

Palpation of the abdomen is performed to assess skin turgor and muscle tone, to determine the size, shape, and position of the abdominal and pelvic organs, and to detect any masses or tenderness. The physician starts with light palpation, which gives information about the abdominal wall and any zones of tenderness, and then progresses to deep palpation to study the internal organs and search for masses. A known area of pain or tenderness is examined last. During abdominal palpation the examiner closely observes the patient's face for signs of distress. Rebound tenderness, a transient stab of pain when the abdomen is pressed and then suddenly released, denotes local or generalized peritoneal irritation. The examiner may look for tenderness in the liver or gallbladder by gentle fist percussion over the right lower ribs or by hooking the fingers of the examining hand under the right costal margin and asking the patient to inhale deeply. Costovertebral angle tenderness occurs in inflammation or infection of the kidney or ureter. The physician may palpate for it at this time by having the patient roll to one side and then the other, or this may already have been done during the examination of the thorax. Inflammation deep in the pelvis can induce painful spasm in muscles originating from pelvic bones and inserting on the femur. Manipulation of the thigh in such cases can elicit significant tenderness (psoas and obturator signs).

skin turgor   muscle tone
acute abdomen   *surgical abdomen*   boardlike rigidity
guarding, spasm, splinting   ticklish
mild epigastric tenderness on deep, firm, vigorous palpation
tenderness and rebound tenderness sharply localized to McBurney point
CVA (costovertebral angle) tenderness   fist percussion
hyperesthesia   jar tenderness
Rovsing sign   Murphy sign
(ilio)psoas sign   obturator sign

Most normal intra-abdominal structures cannot be distinctly felt through the abdominal wall. By vigorous palpation of a very thin subject one can feel parts of the normal liver, spleen, and kidneys, but ordinarily these organs must be enlarged before they can be palpated. A much-distended bladder and a pregnant uterus at or beyond 6-8 weeks' gestation can be felt above the pubic symphysis. No part of the digestive tract can normally be felt, nor can the pancreas, gallbladder, or ureters. In an obese subject even gross abnormalities can escape detection by palpation.

The sigmoid colon is palpable and slightly tender.
hepatomegaly, organomegaly, splenomegaly

The physician systematically goes over the entire abdomen, feeling in each area for possible enlargement of normal structures and looking for masses, pulsations, and tenderness. (Pulsations of the aorta can normally be felt.) To test for enlargement of the liver and spleen, the examiner places a hand just below the right and left costal margin respectively and asks the patient to inhale deeply. Descent of the diaphragm on inspiration will bring an enlarged liver or spleen down into contact with the examining hand. To enhance the sensitivity of the test the physician places the other hand under the patient's ribs on the same side and lifts gently as the patient inhales.

> A soft, smooth, nontender liver edge is palpable 3 fingerbreadths below the right costal margin.
> A spleen tip is palpable.

Any masses detected are thoroughly evaluated as to their size, shape, consistency, attachment to other structures, pulsation, and tenderness. Impacted stool, spasm in the cecum or sigmoid, the sacral promontory, and the tip of a rib are not infrequently mistaken for abnormal masses. Fluid in the abdominal cavity (ascites), if substantial in amount, can be distinguished from obesity by the fact that waves can be set up in it with rhythmic thrusts of the hand. Ballottement over an area filled with fluid can help detect a deep-seated mass or enlarged organ that is not otherwise palpable.

> There is a very firm, irregularly shaped, immobile mass measuring approximately 6 cm in diameter in the left lower quadrant.
>
> ascites   ballotable, ballottement
> fluid wave   free fluid

Percussion, described in the preceding chapter, has some limited applications in the examination of the abdomen. It can be used to measure the liver span (the width of liver dullness between lung and bowel resonances, which is increased when the liver is enlarged) and to distinguish between a solid organ or tumor, which yields a dull or flat note, and bowel distended by gas, which yields a hollow or resonant note. It can also confirm the presence of ascites (free fluid in the peritoneal cavity) by detecting a change in the percussion note as the patient rolls from the supine position to the right or left side (shifting dullness).

> The liver span is 10 cm.   Traube semilinear space
> **percussion note**: dull, flat, hyperresonant, resonant, tympanitic
> meteorism, tympanites   shifting dullness
> Ballance sign

The physician uses auscultation to evaluate the bowel sounds and to listen for bruits. Normal intestinal activity produces characteristic gurgling sounds at intervals of a few seconds. Bowel sounds are reduced or absent in ileus and peritonitis, hyperactive in diarrhea and mechanical intestinal obstruction. Bruits can be heard over narrowed segments of large arteries, including the aorta. Bruits of the renal arteries are listened for through the back, with suitable change in the patient's

For Quick Reference

curdy discharge
cutaneous lesion
CVA (costovertebral angle) tenderness
cyst
cystocele
diagonal conjugate
diaphragm
diastasis recti
dilated veins
direct inguinal hernia
distended abdomen
dull percussion note
endocervical canal
endometrial implants
enlarged organs
enterocele
epididymis
epididymitis
epigastric region
epigastric tenderness
epispadias
everted umbilicus
exquisitely tender prostate
external hemorrhoid
external inguinal ring
external sphincter
fecal impaction
female escutcheon
femoral hernia
fetal heart tones
fetal small parts
fetoscope
FHT (fetal heart tones)
fibroid
fibroma
fibromyoma
fingerbreadths
fishy discharge
fissure in ano
fissures
fist percussion
fistula in ano
fistulous tracts
flat percussion note
fluid in abdominal cavity
fluid wave
Foley catheter
foreskin
foul discharge
free fluid
fundus
genital wart
gentle fist percussion
gestational size
glans penis
green discharge
Grey Turner sign
groin

For Quick Reference

guaiac negative
guarding
gynecologic examination
Hegar sign
heme-negative stool
Hemoccult negative
hemorrhoids
hepatomegaly
herniation
Hesselbach triangle
hockey-stick incision
hydrocele
hyperactive bowel sounds
hyperesthesia
hyperresonant percussion note
hypogastric region
hypospadias
ileostomy
ileus
iliopsoas sign
immobile mass
impacted stool
imperforate hymen
incarcerated hernia
incisional hernia
indirect inguinal hernia
indwelling catheter
infection
inflammation
inguinal adenopathy
inguinal canal
inguinal crease
inguinal fold
inguinal ligament
intact hymen
internal examination
internal hemorrhoid
internal sphincter
intertrigo
intra-abdominal structures
Jacquemeier sign
jar tenderness
kraurosis vulvae
Leopold maneuvers
lesion
linea alba
linea nigra
lithotomy position
liver dullness
liver span
LLQ (left lower quadrant)
LUQ (left upper quadrant)
male escutcheon
marital introitus
McBurney point
meteorism
mons pubis
mons veneris

position. As in the thorax, the presence of both fluid and gas in the abdominal cavity can be demonstrated by hearing a succussion splash with or without a stethoscope when the patient is shaken.

bowel sounds	*silent abdomen*, bowel
peristaltic rushes	bruits, vascular sounds

The abdominal examination concludes with palpation of femoral pulses and an assessment of the groins for dermatitis, enlarged lymph nodes, and hernias. A hernia is the protrusion of some normally contained structure through a weakness or defect in a body wall. Most hernias occur in the groin and contain loops of small intestine. A true inguinal hernia lies above the inguinal ligament, a femoral hernia just below it at the top of the thigh. In the male an indirect inguinal hernia can descend into the scrotum. With recumbency a hernia often reduces; hence the subject is examined for hernias while standing, if possible. The physician positions the examining fingers over each groin in turn and asks the subject to cough vigorously. In examining a male patient, the examiner brings the index finger as close as possible to the external inguinal ring by invaginating a portion of the scrotal skin.

inguinal canal, crease, fold, ligament		pubic symphysis
canal of Nuck	Scarpa triangle	Hesselbach triangle
intertrigo	tinea cruris	
bubo, inguinal adenopathy		visceroptosis
incarcerated, reducible, strangulated hernia		femoral hernia
direct, indirect inguinal hernia		Richter hernia

At this point in the examination of a male patient the physician proceeds to the **external genitalia**. With the patient still standing, the penis and scrotum are examined for dermatitis, ulcers, scars, and other cutaneous lesions. The penis is assessed for developmental anomalies and the foreskin, if present, is retracted for inspection of the glans. The urethra may be milked to express any discharge. The scrotal contents are palpated and any masses, testicular enlargement or deformity, or tenderness is noted. If one or both testicles are not felt in the scrotum, an attempt is made to locate them in the inguinal canals (undescended testis). Scrotal masses are assessed by transillumination. A bright focal light is placed behind and in contact with the scrotum, and the room lights extinguished. A cyst or hydrocele will transmit light; a solid tumor or hernia will not.

glans (penis)	foreskin, prepuce	penile shaft	urethral meatus
male escutcheon	Tanner stage		
crabs, pubic lice	pediculosis, phthiriasis	nits	
epispadias, hypospadias	priapism		
phimosis, paraphimosis	balanitis, posthitis, balanoposthitis	circumcised	

chancre   condyloma acuminatum

scrotal contents   testicle, testis   epididymis

(spermatic) cord   pampiniform plexus

cryptorchism, undescended testicle   anorchia

hydrocele   varicocele

transillumination of the scrotum   orchitis   epididymitis

The examination of this region in the male concludes with a rectal examination. The physician performs a digital rectal examination not only to gather data about the rectum and anus but also to evaluate the pelvic walls and pelvic organs, particularly the prostate in the male, for evidence of tenderness or masses. The patient may stand and bend forward with elbows resting on the examining table, or lie supine or on one side with knees drawn up. The examiner first inspects the anus and perineum for swellings, masses, hemorrhoids, fissures, cutaneous lesions, fistulous tracts, or signs of inflammation. Inserting a gloved and lubricated finger gently into the rectum, the examiner then assesses sphincter tone, notes any tenderness, scarring, or masses in the anal canal, and palpates the interior of the rectum as far as the finger can reach. Any masses, thickening, or fixation of the rectal walls are observed, as well as the amount and consistency of any stool present. The pelvic walls and all structures within reach are palpated, including the prostate and the seminal vesicles. After the finger is withdrawn, any stool, blood, pus, or mucus adhering to the surface of the glove is noted, and a simple chemical test for occult blood may be performed before the glove is discarded.

anoderm, anal verge   external, internal sphincter

hemorrhoid, pile   *sentinel pile*   perineum

external, internal, thrombosed hemorrhoid

anal procidentia, prolapse, protrusion

fissure in ano   fistula in ano

rectal ampulla, pouch   fecal impaction

Blumer rectal shelf

There is a 2 cm stony hard nodule in the left lobe of the prostate.

The prostate is swollen, boggy, and *exquisitely* tender.

2+ prostatic enlargement   BPH (benign prostatic hyperplasia)

The rectal pouch contains a moderate amount of soft brown stool which is guaiac negative.

negative for occult blood

In women the examination of the external and internal genitourinary organs and the rectum and anus is normally performed in the so-called lithotomy position. The subject lies on her back on a specially equipped examining table with her feet in stirrups, her thighs flexed sharply on her abdomen, and her knees spread wide apart. If the subject cannot assume the lithotomy position, the left lateral (Sims) position may be used instead. The physician inspects the pubes and vulva for hair

For Quick Reference

distribution, developmental anomalies, cutaneous lesions, swellings, and signs of inflammation. The urethral meatus and Bartholin and Skene glands are inspected and palpated. The integrity of the pelvic floor is assessed by having the patient bear down while the examiner observes for cystocele (bulging of the urinary bladder through the anterior vaginal wall), rectocele (bulging of the rectum through the posterior vaginal wall), or uterine prolapse. Any vaginal discharge is also observed, and the perineum and anus are examined as noted above for the male.

---

gynecologic, internal, pelvic examination   sterile vaginal examination

female escutcheon   mons pubis, mons veneris   Tanner staging

crabs, pubic lice   pediculosis, phthiriasis   nits

imperforate, intact hymen   marital, parous, virginal introitus

BUS (Bartholin glands, urethra, and Skene glands)

Foley, indwelling catheter

urethral caruncle, pouting   Bartholin abscess, cyst

urethral discharge   bartholinitis, skenitis   kraurosis vulvae

chancre   condyloma acuminatum, genital wart

discharge: brown, curdy, fishy, foul, green, thick, thin, watery, white, yellow

pelvic support   perineum   cystocele, enterocele, rectocele

The physician then inserts a warmed and lubricated bivalve speculum into the vagina, and by spreading its blades and adjusting its position obtains a view of the cervix, fornices, and vaginal walls. Specimens may be taken for cultures or cytologic study at this point. A gynecologist may use a colposcope, which provides bright light and strong magnification, to inspect the cervix. After removing the speculum, the examiner inserts one or two fingers of the dominant hand, gloved and lubricated, into the vagina and places the other hand on the patient's abdomen (bimanual pelvic examination). In this manner the size, shape, and position of the uterus can be assessed, and any masses or tenderness in the pelvic cavity can be detected. Normal uterine adnexa (ovaries, tubes, broad ligaments, round ligaments, and associated blood vessels) can seldom be felt. The physician concludes the examination of the female subject by performing a digital rectal examination. This is done essentially as described for the male, except that the lithotomy position is consistently used, and the examiner inserts one finger in the vagina and another in the rectum at the same time (rectovaginal examination).

---

speculum examination

cervix   endocervical canal   portio vaginalis   squamocolumnar junction

circular sulci   cockscomb deformity   transverse ridges   nabothian cyst

uterus, womb   sacrouterine ligament

anteflexion, anteversion   retroflexion, retroversion

fibroid, fibroma, fibromyoma, myoma   endometrial implants

adnexa, parametria   *chandelier sign*

ovarian cyst   cul-de-sac, pouch of Douglas

If the patient is pregnant the examiner performs certain additional diagnostic procedures. An attempt is made to determine the duration of the pregnancy by a consideration of uterine size. The size and shape of the pelvic outlet are assessed to determine whether it will accommodate the fetus during labor. If the pregnancy is sufficiently advanced, the examiner will attempt to learn by palpation (Leopold maneuvers) the position in which the fetus lies within the uterus. Finally, again if the pregnancy is sufficiently advanced, an attempt is made to hear fetal heart tones by auscultation through the mother's abdomen. A special stethoscope (fetoscope) may be used for this purpose.

The uterus is enlarged to approximately 10 weeks' gestational size.

Chadwick sign   Braxton-Hicks contractions

Jacquemeier sign   placental souffle

Hegar sign   FHT (fetal heart tones)

transverse diameter   diagonal conjugate

fundus   transverse lie

cephalic, breech presentation   fetal small parts

The head is engaged.

For Quick Reference

transverse lie
transverse ridges
Traube semilinear space
traumatic scar
tympanites
tympanitic percussion note
umbilical hernia
umbilicus
undescended testicle
undescended testis (pl. testes)
urethral caruncle
urethral meatus
urethral pouting
uterine adnexa
uterine prolapse
uterus
vagina
vaginal discharge
varices
varicocele
vascular sounds
vigorous palpation
virginal introitus
visceroptosis
visible peristalsis
vulva
watery discharge
white discharge
womb
yellow discharge

Exercises for Chapter 25

Review and Summarize

A. Multiple Choice

___ 1. The lower half of the trunk from the diaphragm to the perineum consists of the
   a. Chest and abdomen.
   b. Abdomen and pelvis.
   c. Pelvis and thorax.
   d. Thorax and extremities.

___ 2. What gland is evaluated on rectal examination of the male patient?
   a. Brunner.
   b. Penis.
   c. Prostate.
   d. Urethral.

___ 3. Percussion over the abdomen is helpful in distinguishing
   a. Bladder spasms.
   b. Gallstones.
   c. Hernias.
   d. Liver span.

___ 4. A solid scrotal mass can be distinguished from a hydrocele by
   a. Auscultation.
   b. Percussion.
   c. Observation.
   d. Transillumination.

B. Fill in the Blank

1. A patient with an ileus or peritonitis would likely have reduced or absent _____ sounds.

2. When a patient lies back-side-down on the table with feet elevated in stirrups, this is the _____

   position.

3. The medical word for bulging of the rectum through the posterior vaginal wall is _____.

4. _____ maneuvers are used to palpate the advanced pregnant uterus to determine fetal

   position.

C. Short Answer

1. What does the physician look for on palpation of the abdomen?

   _____

   _____

   _____

   _____

2. What organs comprise the uterine adnexa?

   _____

   _____

3. Write a short definition of the following terms. If you can, condense the definition into just a few words or a single synonym that you feel more comfortable with.

   a. Supine _____

   b. Umbilicus _____

   c. Varices _____

   d. Stoma _____

   e. Scaphoid _____

   f. Panniculus _____

   g. Cholecystectomy _____

   h. Organomegaly _____

   i. Peristalsis _____

   j. Balanitis _____

   k. Cryptorchism _____

   l. Epididymitis _____

   m. Lithotomy _____

   n. Escutcheon _____

o. Pediculosis _____

p. Fibroid _____

q. Sphincter _____

r. Piles _____

Pause and Reflect

Draw a mind map for each of the five areas of this examination: abdomen, groins, rectum, anus, and genitalia. For each area, list three to five examination techniques or maneuvers. For each of these, list up to five related findings from the list of terms that accompanies this chapter.

Relate and Remember

Create a visual representation of the physical examination of this area of the body. You may use a drawing, flow chart, graph, diagram, or metaphorical illustration. Explain, if necessary, how the visual representation relates to your exam.

Collaborate and Share

As a group, combine your knowledge of conditions affecting the abdomen, groins, rectum, anus, and genitalia. List as many conditions as you can based on your personal experience or studies, but without referring to the textbook. Share your list with the rest of the class.

_____

_____

_____

_____

_____

_____

_____

_____

Explain and Learn

Turn to the person next to you (or behind or in front of you), and share with each other one important piece of information you got from this chapter. Also share how you might use this information in your life or in your work. If you have a question that wasn't answered in the chapter, share that as well. If your partner doesn't have the answer, ask your instructor.

Relax and Play

1. After reviewing the chapter as a class or in small groups, the instructor will announce "Go," and individual class members will "pop up" and call out one important fact learned, already known, or remembered about a topic or section in this chapter.

2. Select 10 to 20 words or phrases from the word list in this chapter and create a word search puzzle. Rather than list the words you've chosen, however, list the definitions as clues. Copy the puzzles to share with the rest of the class. Students must first determine which word goes with the definition before finding it in the puzzle.

Generalize and Apply

Write on a 3" x 5" card a statement of something you learned and how you think this information will help you or a question as yet unanswered. You must turn this card in to the instructor as your "ticket out" of class.

Compare and Contrast

1. What is the difference between an *inguinal hernia* and a *femoral hernia*?

_____

_____

_____

_____

2. What's the distinction between *tenderness* and *pain*? How are they similar?

_____

_____

_____

_____

Extrapolate and Project

It can be difficult to diagnose the cause of abdominal pain because more than a hundred conditions affecting various parts of the body can produce abdominal pain. Speculate on the causes of abdominal pain that might originate outside of the abdominal and pelvic organs.

_____

_____

_____

_____

_____

_____

_____

_____

_____

_____

_____

_____

_____

_____

26

Examination of the Back and Extremities

The physician examines the back and extremities to detect abnormalities of the skin and subcutaneous tissues in these regions, injuries and diseases of the musculoskeletal system, disorders of circulation, and evidence of central or peripheral nervous system disease. The examinations of the skin, bones, joints, muscles, and peripheral circulation are described in this chapter, and of the nervous system in the next. In actual practice, however, the physician generally investigates one bodily region at a time rather than one system at a time.

> The back is straight and flexible and the extremities show no tremor, edema, cyanosis, or clubbing.

The back and extremities are examined according to whatever routine the physician finds most expedient, with suitable modifications for the patient's condition and ability to cooperate. Clothing is removed as needed for the examination of each region, and the patient is positioned for maximum comfort. A full orthopedic examination requires considerable cooperation from the patient in assuming various positions and performing various movements. The history and physical findings influence the scope and thoroughness of the examination in that some special procedures are applied only when indicated.

> distal, proximal   palmar, plantar, volar
> articular, periarticular   dorsal, ventral

Inspection and palpation of the skin are carried out as described in previous chapters. The hands and feet are examined particularly for cutaneous lesions, and the appearance of the nails is carefully noted. The physician looks for clubbing of fingers or toes, seen in chronic pulmonary disease and certain other conditions, and observes the nail beds for pallor or cyanosis. Painless swelling of the ankles and feet (dependent edema), which can indicate cardiac failure, renal disease, protein deficiency, or venous obstruction, is noted and graded. Pitting refers to the formation of pits or indentations when the fingers are pressed into edematous tissue. The girth of a swollen extremity is determined with a tape measure and compared to the other side measured at the same level.

The peripheral circulation is assessed in several ways. Blood flow in major arteries is determined by palpation and grading of pulses, with comparison of the two sides. Suspicious regions can be auscultated for bruits caused by arterial

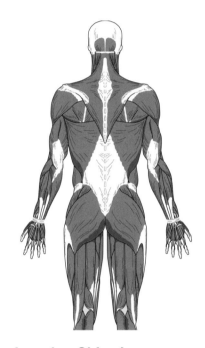

Learning Objectives

After careful study of this chapter, you should be able to:

Identify findings and conditions revealed on inspection and palpation of the skin.

Explain methods of assessment of the peripheral circulation.

Describe three ways in which joint range of motion can be determined.

Identify terms related to examination of the bones and muscles.

Describe procedures related to the examination of the back.

Name and define tests of the back and extremities.

Match orthopedic exam findings with a particular body region or system.

For Quick Reference

AC (acromioclavicular) joint
Ace bandage; wrapping
Ace splint
acrocyanosis
acromegaly
acropachy
active and passive range of motion
Adson test
AK (above knee) amputation
Allen test
anatomic snuffbox
ankylosing spondylitis
anserine bursitis
antalgic gait
Apley test
apraxic gait
arachnodactyly
arthroplasty
ataxic gait
atrophy
avulsion fracture
Baker cyst
Bancroft sign
Beau lines
BK (below knee) amputation
Bouchard nodes
boutonnière deformity
brawny edema
Brodie test
buffalo hump
bursting-type laceration
Calloway test
capillary circulation
capillary refill
carpal tunnel
cervical spondylosis
circulation compromise
claw hand
clubbing of extremities
cockup splint
concave nails
Corrigan pulse
coxa valga
coxa vara
Cozen test
crepitus
cubitus valgus
cyanosis of extremities
dependent edema
deQuervain disease
dermatitis
dextroscoliosis
dicrotic pulse
DIP (distal interphalangeal) joint
dorsalis pedis pulse
dorsiflexion
dowager's hump
drawer sign

---

acropachy, scleroderma   palmar erythema   acrocyanosis
ganglion   tophus   Osler nodes   Janeway spots
epitrochlear nodes   clubbing
cuticle   nail bed   eponychium   lunula   Beau lines
leukonychia, koilonychia, paronychia
onchyolysis, onychogryposis, onychophytosis
nails: concave, drumstick, dystrophic, floating, fluted, hippocratic, parrot-beak, pitted, serpent-head, spoon
splinter hemorrhage   subungual hematoma
edema: brawny, dependent, pedal, pitting, pretibial   2+ pitting edema
Bancroft, Homans, Lowenberg sign
Both calves measure 36.5 cm, 4 fingerbreadths below the lower poles of the patellae.
There is a 2 cm indolent ulcer just anterior to the right medial malleolus
pulse: popliteal, radial, ulnar, brachial   pedal pulses
dorsalis pedis, posterior tibial pulse   pulsus alternans
pulsus bisferiens, celer, parvus, tardus   capillary refill
Corrigan, dicrotic, thready, water-hammer pulse   nail-bed cyanosis
Quincke capillary pulse   circulation, vascular *compromise*
Allen test   bruit
Adson test   arteriovenous fistula
subclavian steal
greater, lesser saphenous system   communicating veins, feeders
bilateral saphenous varices without evidence of dermatitis or venous stasis
Perthes, tourniquet, Trendelenburg test   phlegmasia alba dolens
lymphedema   phlegmasia cerulea dolens

---

narrowing or compression or by arteriovenous fistula. Capillary circulation can be tested by observing the rate at which a compressed area, such as a nail bed, refills (becomes pink again) when the pressure is released. In the Allen test, the physician assesses circulation in the hand by watching for flushing after release of a compressed radial or ulnar artery. In the Adson test for compression of the subclavian artery at the thoracic outlet, the physician palpates for changes in the radial pulse while the subject turns the head to the opposite side and inhales deeply. The examiner looks for varicose (dilated and tortuous) veins, particularly in the lower extremities. When saphenous varices are present, the Trendelenburg and Brodie tests, which require application of a tourniquet to the thigh, may be used to determine the competence of venous valves and the patency of the deep venous channels.

Having considered the skin and the circulation, the examiner assesses the bones, joints, muscles, and other connective and supporting structures, looking for any developmental or traumatic deformities not previously noted and any evidence of generalized conditions such as muscle wasting or weakness, stiffness, or tremors. The terms *varus* and *valgus* refer to abnormal deviations in joints of the extremities. In a varus deformity, the bone distal to the affected joint is deviated inward; hence *genu varum* means *bowleg*. Valgus is outward deviation of the distal bone; hence *genu valgum* means *knock-knee*.

abduction extension dorsiflexion inversion

adduction flexion plantar flexion eversion

circumduction internal rotation external rotation

valgus, varus

arthroscopy scars arthroplasty

Taylor brace cockup splint

Ace bandage, cast, splint, wrapping prosthesis

atrophy, wasting weakness

contracture immobility

micromelia acromegaly

DIP (distal interphalangeal) PIP (proximal interphalangeal)

MCP (metacarpophalangeal)

ulnar deviation and subluxation of the metacarpophalangeal joints of the right hand

Heberden nodes, Bouchard nodes, Haygarth nodes

arachnodactyly, spider fingers, Marfan syndrome

mallet finger boutonnière, swan-neck deformity

claw, spade hand Dupuytren contracture

trigger finger stenosing tenosynovitis, deQuervain disease

anatomic snuffbox silver fork deformity

flail arm lateral, medial epicondyle

tennis elbow, lateral epicondylitis increased carrying angle, cubitus valgus

olecranon bursitis

rotator cuff supraspinatus tendon

frozen shoulder winged scapula

AC (acromioclavicular) joint

hammer toe hallux valgus

bunion, callus, corn, soft corn, clavum

pes cavus, equinus, planus *intoeing, toeing in*

talipes calcaneovalgus, equinovarus

AK (above knee), BK (below knee) **amputation**

genu recurvatum, valgum, varum internal derangement of the knee

Baker cyst anserine, prepatellar bursitis

hamstrings *joint mice*

quadriceps atrophy, wasting

greater, lesser trochanter infragluteal crease

gluteus intergluteal cleft

buttocks, nates coxa valga, vara

leg length discrepancy

strength point tenderness, *trigger point*

tone atrophy

For Quick Reference

drumstick nails
duck waddle
Dugas test
Dupuytren contracture
dystrophic nails
epitrochlear nodes
extravasated blood
fabere test
fadir test
fasciitis
festinating gait
flail arm
floating nails
fluted nails
frozen shoulder
full-thickness burn
Gaenslen test
genu valgum
genu varum
genu recurvatum
glue-footed gait
hallux valgus
Hamilton ruler test
hammer toe
hamstrings
Haygarth nodes
Heberden nodes
hemarthrosis
hematoma formation
hemiplegic gait
hippocratic nails
Homans sign
hysterical gait
iliac crest
indolent ulcer
infragluteal crease
instability on stress testing
intergluteal cleft
Janeway spots
Jobe test
joint mice
koilonychia
kyphosis
Lachman test
Lasegue test
lateral epicondylitis
latissimus dorsi
leg length discrepancy
leukonychia
levoscoliosis
lordosis
loss of normal lordotic curve
Lowenberg sign
lumbar laminectomy scar
lymphedema
mallet finger
Marfan syndrome
McMurray test

For Quick Reference

MCP (metacarpophalangeal) joint
mediolateral stress
meningocele
micromelia
muscle wasting
mushy edema
myofasciitis
myofibrositis
myositis
nail-bed cyanosis
olecranon bursitis
onychogryposis
onycholysis
onychophytosis
Osler nodes
O'Brien test
palindromic rheumatism
palmar erythema
paraspinal muscles
paravertebral muscles
paronychia
parrot-beak nails
partial-thickness burn
Patrick test
pedal edema
peripheral circulation
Perthes test
pes cavus
pes equinus
pes planus
Phalen test
phlegmasia alba dolens
phlegmasia cerulea dolens
pilonidal cyst
pilonidal dimple
pilonidal sinus
pilonidal tract
PIP (proximal interphalangeal) joint
pitted nails
pitting edema
plantar flexion
point tenderness
poker spine
polyarthritis
polyarthropathy
popliteal pulse
posterior tibial pulse
prepatellar bursitis
pretibial edema
propulsion gait
pseudarthrosis
pulsus alternans
pulsus bisferiens
pulsus celer
pulsus parvus
pulsus tardus
quadriceps atrophy
Quincke capillary pulse

spasm   fasciitis, myofasciitis, myositis
myofibrositis
clicking, crepitus, popping, rubbing, snapping
polyarthritis, polyarthropathy   palindromic rheumatism
ankylosis, pseudarthrosis   hemarthrosis
effusion   laxity, instability   stress testing

Specific procedures and techniques are applied for each anatomic region, but the same basic principles are followed for all regions. Besides inspecting and palpating, the physician puts joints through a passive range of motion and has the patient put them through an active range of motion, with or without resistance by the examiner. Muscles are assessed for development, bilateral symmetry, strength, tone, and spasm or tenderness. Bones are assessed for deformity, masses, or tenderness. A joint is not simply the place where two bones are hooked together but a complex structure with highly specialized tissues, subject to many injuries and diseases. The physician examines joints for swelling, stiffness, thickening of synovial membranes, fluid, tenderness, and instability. The range of movement in a joint can be quantified with a goniometer, a simple device consisting of two arms connected at a movable joint, with a scale that reads in degrees of rotation.

In examining an injured extremity the physician notes any swelling, deformity, cutaneous trauma, ecchymosis, or hematoma formation. The age of subcutaneous hemorrhage can be judged by its color. Muscular and skeletal structures are palpated for tenderness, spasm, deformity, or discontinuity, and active and passive ranges of motion are checked. Joints are palpated for crepitus or effusion and tested by manipulation for ligamentous laxity. The circulation and sensation of the part are also carefully evaluated.

There is a diffuse zone of mushy edema over the anterior talofibular ligament with faint ecchymosis, slight tenderness to palpation and manipulation, but no deformity, crepitus, instability on stress testing, or impairment of circulation or sensation.

fracture   dislocation, luxation   subluxation
separation   sprain, strain
open wound   clean, contaminated, contused
abrasion, scrape, scratch, gouge   avulsion
incised wound, cut   puncture   tissue defect
laceration   stellate, bursting-type laceration
closed wound   bruise, contusion
burn, scald   frostbite, chilblain, pernio
full-thickness, partial-thickness burn
ecchymosis, extravasated blood, hematoma
epitrochlear nodes

The back is examined first with the subject standing and facing away from the examiner. Any spinal curvature or developmental deformities are noted, as well as

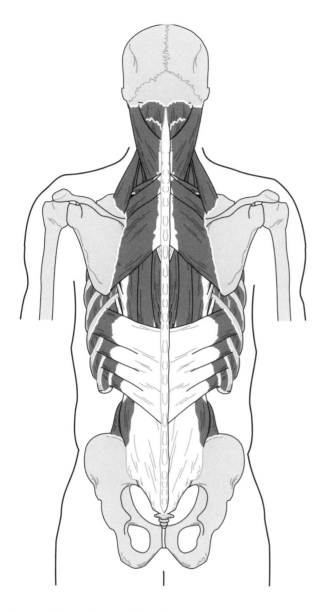

any surgical scars. The heights of the iliac crests are compared as a rough test of leg length equality. The spinous processes of the vertebrae, the sacroiliac joints, and the sciatic notches are assessed by palpation for tenderness, the muscles for tenderness and spasm. The examiner notes the range of spinal movements as the subject bends forward, backward, and to the sides. The subject then lies supine (face up) on the examining table and the physician tests for disorders of the sacroiliac and hip joints and for sciatic nerve irritation by manipulation of the lower extremities. Further examinations may be conducted with the subject prone (face down). The mobility of the subject in getting on and off the examining table is noted.

The shoulders, elbows, wrists, knuckles, knees, and ankles are examined by a set of standard procedures appropriate to each region, and special tests are applied for the assessment of any abnormalities noted. The patient's stance and gait are also observed for evidence of listing or limping due to weakness, spasm, or pain. Abnormalities of stance and gait often have neurologic rather than orthopedic implications.

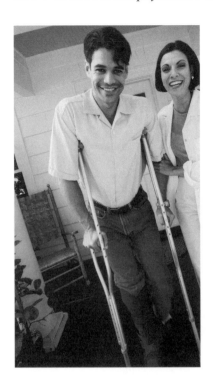

spine, spinal column, vertebral column   spinous processes

sacroiliac joints

paraspinal muscles, paravertebral muscles   sciatic notch

buffalo hump, dowager's hump   kyphosis, lordosis, scoliosis

dextroscoliosis, levoscoliosis, rotoscoliosis   Scheuermann disease

cervical spondylosis   torticollis, wryneck

ankylosing spondylitis   poker spine

loss of normal lordotic curve   latissimus dorsi

spina bifida, meningocele   lumbar laminectomy scar

pilonidal cyst, dimple, sinus, tract

active and passive range of motion

Speed, O'Brien, Jobe test

The elbow is limited to 160° of extension and 75° of flexion.

hand grip   carpal, tarsal tunnel

Phalen, Tinel test   Cozen test

Hamilton ruler test   Calloway, Dugas test   Yergason test

drawer sign   Lachman, Apley, McMurray test

Mediolateral stress reveals no instability.

duck waddle

Ballottement of the patella reveals no effusion.

Both quadriceps muscles measure 47 cm, 4 fingerbreadths above the patellae.

sciatic nerve stretch

Lasegue, Gaenslen, Trendelenburg, Patrick test   *fabere, fadir* test

varus, valgus stress   goniometer

posture, stance, station

gait: antalgic, apraxic, ataxic, festinating, glue-footed, hemiplegic, hysterical, propulsion, scissors, shuffling, spastic, steppage, Trendelenburg, waddling

Exercises for Chapter 26

Review and Summarize

A. Multiple Choice

___ 1. Varices are
   a. Dilated veins.
   b. Healing scabs.
   c. Old abscesses.
   d. Deep-seated scars.

___ 2. A patient with bowlegs suffers from
   a. Plantar flexion.
   b. Dorsiflexion.
   c. Genu valgum.
   d. Genu varum.

___ 3. The iliac crest heights are compared to check for
   a. Uniform skin coloration.
   b. Equal leg lengths.
   c. Fractures or dislocations.
   d. Tumors or other lesions.

B. Fill in the Blank

1. _____ range of motion is carried out when the physician, not the patient, puts the joints through a series of movements.

2. Range of motion in a joint can be determined with an instrument that reads degrees of rotation, called a(n)

   _____.

3. Swelling of the ankles and feet while in the legs are in the dependent position is known as dependent

   _____.

C. Short Answer

1. How is the age of a subcutaneous hemorrhage judged?

2. Describe the assessment of peripheral circulation.

_____

_____

_____

_____

_____

_____

_____

3. Write a short definition of the following terms. If you can, condense the definition into just a few words or a single synonym that you feel more comfortable with.

a. Dorsal_____

b. Ventral _____

c. Plantar _____

d. Volar_____

e. Palmar _____

f. Proximal_____

g. Distal _____

h. Tortuous_____

i. Clubbing _____

j. Pedal _____

k. Abduction _____

l. Adduction _____

m. Circumduction_____

n. Acromegaly_____

o. Wasting _____

p. Atrophy _____

Pause and Reflect

Type on a separate sheet or handwrite below the physical examination of your own back and extremities, using the criteria described in this chapter. Be sure to indicate pertinent negatives as well as positive findings.

_____

_____

_____

_____

_____

_____

_____

Relate and Remember

Think of a metaphor that completes this statement: The extremities are like a(n) _____. Use a visual or a verbal metaphor. You may fill in the blank with the name of an object or draw (or cut out of a magazine) a picture representing one or more important points. Explain your choice.

_____

_____

_____

_____

_____

_____

_____

_____

Collaborate and Share

Role-play a doctor in an emergency room setting, performing a physical examination of the back and extremities for a patient who has been in an automobile accident. Have the doctor narrate the examination techniques and findings. Have another student record the findings. Switch roles so that each student gets a turn as physician, patient, and recorder. Transcribe the notes you took as recorder.

Explain and Learn

Make an outline for this chapter, assigning a heading for each paragraph. List one to five important facts as subheadings. Explain your choices.

_____

_____

_____

_____

_____

_____

_____

_____

_____

_____

_____

_____

_____

_____

_____

Relax and Play

1. With students divided into groups, each group selects a different game show ("Who Wants to be a Millionaire," "Jeopardy," "Hollywood Squares," etc.) and creates an "episode" using questions and answers related to this chapter. The games are presented using contestants from other groups. The class then votes on the best game presented.

2. Fold a blank piece of paper in half three times so that when unfolded there are eight squares. Write one thing you learned in each square. Move around the room, asking other students to define or explain an item on your sheet. That student then signs the square. The student who gets all eight squares signed first wins.

Generalize and Apply

Draw a mind map representing the examination of the back and extremities. In the secondary ring of circles list the skin, peripheral circulation, and bones/joints/muscles. In the next ring, list the methods by which each of these is assessed. In the third ring, list 5 to 10 findings for each of these methods. Use as many terms as you can from the word list that accompanies this chapter.

Compare and Contrast

What is the difference between *active* and *passive* range of motion? With a partner, demonstrate each technique.

_____

_____

_____

_____

Extrapolate and Project

Osteoporosis leads to bone fragility and increased susceptibility to fractures of the hip, spine, and wrist, especially in women. Investigate osteoporosis to learn what causes it, how it is diagnosed, and what treatments are currently available. Use your textbooks and other outside resources as necessary. Summarize your findings below.

_____

_____

_____

_____

_____

_____

_____

_____

_____

_____

_____

27

The Neurologic Examination

The examination of the central and peripheral nervous systems, like that of the heart, consists almost exclusively of tests of function. Many of these tests require the cooperation of the patient. However, the more urgent the need for a neurologic exam, the less capable may the patient be to cooperate. The extreme example is the comatose patient, whose life may depend on prompt and accurate diagnosis but who cannot cooperate at all. The basic neurologic examination is augmented by special procedures as history and findings direct.

> Neurologic exam reveals no gross sensory or motor deficits.
>
> brain stem　　　pons　　　midbrain

Most parts of the neurologic examination are carried out on a regional basis and interspersed with examinations of other systems. In analyzing and recording findings, however, the physician classifies them according to anatomic and functional divisions of the nervous system. The central nervous system (CNS) comprises the brain and spinal cord; the peripheral nervous system, the cranial and spinal nerves. Peripheral nerve fibers are either motor (efferent) fibers carrying impulses to muscles, or sensory (afferent) fibers carrying impulses to the spinal cord or brain stem. Both kinds of fibers are often combined in a single nerve trunk.

The physician tests sensory functions by stimulating appropriate receptors and noting the subject's responses. Motor functions are tested by observing the subject's ability to perform certain actions. Even in an unconscious patient, testing the deep tendon reflexes enables the examiner to assess the integrity of the spinal reflex arcs, which consist of both sensory (stretch receptor) and motor nerve fibers. But evaluation of complex voluntary movements and muscle coordination requires the conscious collaboration of the patient. Assessment of cerebral functions (memory, orientation, thinking capacity, mood) is described in the next chapter.

If the patient is stuporous or unconscious, the physician tries to determine the degree of central nervous system depression by noting the size and reactivity of the pupils, the rate and rhythm of breathing, the response to noxious stimuli such as loud noises and firm pressure over bony prominences, and the presence of certain primitive reflexes such as the corneal and gag reflex. In the doll's eye maneuver, the examiner rotates the patient's head from side to side and notes the effect on eye position. Normally the eyes rotate in a direction opposite to that in which the head is moved, tending to maintain the same direction of gaze (oculocephalic reflex). Failure of the eyes to rotate around their own vertical axes during this maneuver indicates brain stem damage.

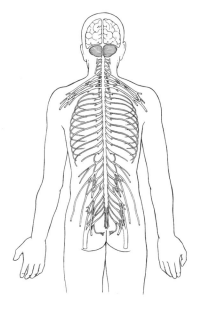

Learning Objectives

After careful study of this chapter, you should be able to:

Name the anatomic and functional divisions of the nervous system.

Discuss the exam of the unconscious patient.

List the 12 pairs of cranial nerves and describe tests of their function.

Define deep tendon, superficial, and pathologic reflexes, giving an example of each.

Give four examples of tests of motor coordination.

Match terms describing abnormal movements with their definitions.

Describe the components of a complete sensory examination.

For Quick Reference

comatose, unconscious, unresponsive   Glasgow coma score

postictal state   catalepsy

corneal, gag reflex   doll's eye maneuver

The twelve pairs of **cranial nerves** emanate from the brain stem and pass to structures in the head and neck. The first pair of cranial nerves (olfactory) are not routinely tested but, as noted in Chapter 21, the sense of smell can be evaluated by asking the subject to identify common substances (soap, tobacco) by their odors. The second pair (optic) are inspected during the funduscopic examination and their function is checked through vision testing (Chapter 19). The third, fourth, and sixth pairs (oculomotor, trochlear, and abducens) control ocular movements (Chapter 19). The fifth pair (trigeminal) supply the face with motor and sensory branches. They are tested by noting the strength of jaw clenching and the sensitivity of the facial skin in various areas to gentle pinprick. The seventh pair (facial) innervate the muscles of the face and are tested by having the patient grimace, purse the lips, wrinkle the forehead, close the eyes tightly, and so on (Chapter 18). The sense of taste on the anterior two-thirds of the tongue is also supplied by the seventh pair. This can be tested by touching the tongue with a drop of salt or sugar solution or vinegar. The eighth pair (vestibulocochlear) are the nerves of hearing and equilibrium (Chapter 20). Testing the pharyngeal (gag) reflex assesses both the ninth pair (glossopharyngeal), which carry the afferent side of this reflex arc (as well as taste afferents from the posterior third of the tongue), and the tenth (vagus), which carry the efferent side. The vagus innervates the muscles of the soft palate as well as those involved in swallowing and speech. The eleventh pair (spinal accessory) send motor fibers to the sternocleidomastoid muscles at the sides of the neck. These are tested by having the subject rotate the head against a resisting hand placed alongside the chin. The twelfth pair (hypoglossal) innervate the tongue and are tested by assessing the patient's ability to protrude the tongue.

Cranial nerves II through XII are intact.

bulbar, pseudobulbar palsy   jaw jerk

Bell palsy   Bell phenomenon

Horner syndrome   Adie pupil

Argyll Robertson pupil   Marcus Gunn pupil

The **spinal nerves** emerge from the spinal cord in pairs, one right and one left, and supply the body from the occiput downward with sensory and motor fibers. A pair of spinal nerves is named from the vertebra above which (cervical region) or below which (other regions) it emerges. Thus the L2 pair emerge below the second lumbar vertebra. Sensory nerve endings in the skin are distributed in segments called dermatomes, each corresponding to a pair of spinal nerves. Sensory and motor fibers to the limbs pass through complicated systems of branching and interconnection (brachial and lumbar plexuses) before forming the main nerve trunks of the upper and lower extremities. The entire skin surface can be mapped as to the segmental origin of its sensory supply, and likewise the spinal segment or segments innervating each muscle are known. With this anatomical knowledge in hand, the physician can localize and characterize lesions of the spinal cord and peripheral nerves by precise study of sensory and motor deficits. In addition, lesions of the brain can be localized by their effect on coordination, stereognosis, and other complex motor and sensory functions.

The examiner obtains some information about the motor system from the first view of the patient, and gains more as the examination proceeds. Generalized weakness, hemiparesis, disturbances of gait, posture, or speech, and abnormal movements such as tics and tremors are readily observed. The orthopedic examination provides data about muscle mass, strength, tone, and control. Paralyzed or disused muscles eventually undergo contracture and atrophy. Paralysis due to peripheral (lower motor neuron) disease is flaccid (muscles soft and limp). Paralysis due to a cerebral (upper motor neuron) lesion is spastic (muscles tight, with rigid or jerky resistance to movement by the examiner) because of uninterrupted, but no longer efficacious, postural and checking signals from the basal ganglia of the brain.

In neurology, the term *reflex* refers to a muscular contraction in response to some stimulus, such as tapping the patellar tendon. For a reflex to occur, both sensory and motor limbs of the reflex arc must be intact. A deep tendon reflex, such as the familiar knee jerk, is elicited by tapping the tendon smartly with a rubber reflex hammer. For some tendons, such as that of the biceps brachii, the examiner may place a thumb firmly over the tendon and then strike the thumb with the hammer. This doesn't feel very good but it vastly improves the accuracy of aim. The examiner tests selected tendons (at a minimum, the biceps and triceps in the arm and the patellar and calcaneal in the leg) and notes the quality and strength of responses, comparing right and left. Normally a sudden stretch of a voluntary muscle tendon elicits a prompt, brisk, transitory contraction of the muscle. In lower motor neuron

For Quick Reference

neuralgia
neuritis
neuromuscular irritability
nuchal rigidity
oculocephalic reflex
Oppenheim reflex
overshooting
palmomental reflex
palsy
paralysis
paresis
patellar clonus
patellar reflex
pathologic reflex
peripheral neuropathy
pinprick
pinwheel
polyneuritis
pons
postictal state
postural tremor
proprioception
propulsion gait
pseudobulbar palsy
pyramidal signs
quadriceps reflex
radiculitis
radiculopathy
ratchet rigidity
resting tremor
risus sardonicus
root signs
scissors gait
Semmes-Weinstein monofilament
sensory deficit
sensory loss
shuffling gait
spastic gait
spastic paralysis
spinal nerves
steppage gait
stereognosis
Stewart-(Gordon) Holmes sign
stocking anesthesia
stuporous
tetany
tic
topognosis
Trendelenburg gait
triceps reflex
tripod sign
Trousseau sign
twitch
two-point discrimination
unconscious
unresponsive
upgoing Babinskis
vibratory sense

lesions the reflexes are reduced or absent. In upper motor neuron lesions the reflexes are not only unimpaired but exaggerated. Besides deep tendon reflexes, superficial or cutaneous reflexes yield information about peripheral sensory and motor nerves. These include the abdominal and cremasteric reflexes. Abdominal reflexes, elicited by stroking the relaxed abdomen, cause contraction of abdominal wall muscles, with movement of the umbilicus toward the area stroked. The cremasteric reflex causes the testicle to draw up when the physician strokes the skin of the inner thigh.

DTR (deep tendon reflex)	areflexia, hyperreflexia, hyporeflexia

reflex: Achilles, biceps, brachioradialis, patellar, quadriceps, triceps

ankle, knee jerk   Jendrassik maneuver

abdominal, anal, cremasteric reflex   *root signs*

Certain reflexes are seen only with upper motor neuron damage (pathologic reflexes). These include the Babinski (upward deviation of the great toe on stroking the sole of the foot), the Hoffman (twitching of the thumb when the middle finger is snapped), and the palmomental (twitching of the chin on stimulation of the palm of the hand).

corticospinal, pyramidal, long tract signs   pathologic reflex

patellar clonus, ankle clonus

Babinski, plantar reflex   Babinskis are *downgoing, upgoing*

Wartenberg reflex   Hoffman reflex   Chaddock reflex   Oppenheim reflex

Gordon reflex   glabellar sign   Myerson sign   grasp reflex

Mayer reflex   palmomental reflex

Motor coordination is tested by having the patient perform complex actions such as touching the nose with the eyes closed, running one heel up and down the opposite shin while recumbent, and making rapidly alternating movements with both hands. In the Gordon Holmes test, the patient is asked to pull with one fist against the physician's resistance in such a way that, if coordination is abnormal, the physician's sudden release of resistance will result in the fist striking the patient's own face. (The physician, however, prevents this.)

adiadochokinesis, dysdiadochokinesis   ataxia, incoordination

heel-to-shin test   finger-to-nose test

checking   *overshooting*

decomposition of movement   Stewart-(Gordon) Holmes sign

apraxia, dyspraxia   dysmetria, dyssynergia

associated movements

Abnormal movements vary from fine, ineffectual twitches of a few muscle fibers (fasciculations) to violent thrusting or hurling movements of the whole body.

Tremors can be coarse or fine, local or generalized; they may be worse at rest (resting tremor), with purposeful movement (intention tremor), or with position-holding (postural tremor). Asterixis is a coarse, flapping tremor that occurs when the patient attempts to hold the hands steady with palms down. Chorea denotes sudden, brief, involuntary jerking movements of the face or limbs; athetosis is a slow, continuous writhing. Often these two occur together.

adventitious movements   myoclonus   myokymia

tetany   carpopedal spasm

hemiballismus   tic, twitch, habit spasm

chorea, athetosis   fasciculation, fibrillation

The physician performs a basic sensory examination by noting the subject's ability to detect light touch (as from a soft brush or a wisp of cotton) and superficial pain (from a gentle pinprick) over various parts of the body surface, always comparing right and left. Nylon monofilaments of various calibers, which buckle at reproducible pressures, can be used to quantify cutaneous sensory loss. Their principal application is in grading diabetic neuropathy of the feet. Sensitivity to temperature can be tested by applying cool and warm metal discs, or test tubes containing cool and warm water, to the skin. Vibratory sense is tested by placing the shank of a vibrating tuning fork against a superficially lying bone, such as a knuckle or shin. Proprioception is a form of sensation by which the brain monitors the position and degree of stretch of voluntary muscles in the trunk and limbs. It is important for both balance sense and coordination. Proprioception can be tested by asking the patient to report the position in which fingers or toes are placed by the examiner.

tactile, touch   pain, temperature, and tactile

anesthesia, hyperesthesia, hyp(o)esthesia

10 g Semmes-Weinstein monofilament

glove, stocking anesthesia   kinesthesia

pinprick, pinwheel   vibratory sense

proprioception   meralgia paresthetica

Other sensory modalities that are tested in selected cases are two-point discrimination (the ability to distinguish two adjacent, simultaneous pinpricks), stereognosis (the ability to identify objects solely by feeling them), and graphesthesia (the ability to recognize letters or numbers traced on the skin).

two-point discrimination   barognosis

topognosis   stereognosis   graphesthesia

Meningitis (inflammation of the covering membranes of the brain and spinal cord) is often accompanied by painful spasm of paraspinal and leg muscles.

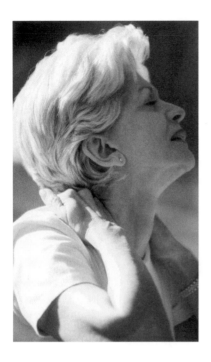

Marked stiffness of the neck (nuchal rigidity) is a cardinal finding in meningitis. In addition, two signs are often present. The Kernig sign is inability of the knee to be extended when the hip is flexed, because of spasm. The Brudzinski sign is involuntary flexion of the hips and knees when the neck is flexed by the examiner.

nuchal rigidity	Kernig sign	Brudzinski sign

Tetany, a hyperirritable state of the neuromuscular system, can be induced by various drugs and metabolic states, particularly hypocalcemia. Signs of tetany are involuntary muscle twitches and spasms, including carpopedal spasm and risus sardonicus, and the Trousseau and Chvostek signs. The Chvostek sign is spastic contraction of facial muscles induced by tapping over the facial nerve in front of the ear. The Trousseau sign is spastic contraction of wrist and forearm muscles induced by inflation of a sphygmomanometer cuff placed about the arm above systolic pressure.

neuromuscular irritability	tetany
carpopedal spasm	risus sardonicus
Chvostek sign	Trousseau sign

Exercises for Chapter 27

Review and Summarize

A. Multiple Choice

___ 1. How many pair of cranial nerves exist in the human body?
   a. 6.
   b. 8.
   c. 10.
   d. 12.

___ 2. Sensory nerve endings are distributed in segments in the skin known as
   a. Reflexes.
   b. Peripheral nerves.
   c. Motor nerves.
   d. Dermatomes.

___ 3. The twitching of muscle fibers is called (Mark two.)
   a. Ventriculation.
   b. Fasciculation.
   c. Vesiculation.
   d. Fibrillation.

___ 4. The ability to identify objects by touch only is known as
   a. Graphesthesia.
   b. Two-point discrimination.
   c. Stereognosis.
   d. Vibratory sense.

B. Fill in the Blank

1. The brain and _____ comprise the central nervous system.

2. A muscular contraction in response to a stimulus is called a(n) _____.

3. The Babinski, Hoffman, and palmomental are all examples of _____ reflexes.

4. Tremors may be categorized as postural, intention, or _____.

C. Short Answer

1. How does the physician assess neurologic status on physical examination of an unconscious patient?

   _____

   _____

   _____

   _____

   _____

2. Describe the oculocephalic reflex.

   _____

   _____

   _____

3. Why is the orthopedic examination important in evaluating the nervous system?

   _____

   _____

   _____

4. Write a short definition of the following terms. If you can, condense the definition into just a few words or a single synonym that you feel more comfortable with.

   a. Catalepsy_____

   b. Bulbar palsy _____

   c. Radiculopathy _____

   d. Dyskinesia_____

   e. Decorticate _____

   f. Apraxia _____

   g. Ataxia _____

h. Afferent _____

i. Antalgic gait _____

j. Cremasteric _____

k. Pyramidal signs _____

l. Palmomental _____

m Dysdiadochokinesis _____

n. Dyssynergia _____

o. Kinesthesia_____

p. Nuchal _____

q. Tetany _____

Pause and Reflect

Have you ever known anyone who suffered from a condition affecting the neurologic system? What symptoms did they have? Go through the chapter and locate the symptoms associated with this condition and underline them. Then circle the tests associated with these symptoms.

Relate and Remember

Take a sheet of paper and draw lines to create four columns, labeled A through D. List five important things to remember about the chapter. Put these in column A. In column B, next to each of the items to remember, write the name of an object that might help you to remember the fact. In column C, write the name of a place that might help you to remember the fact. In column D, write a description of a visual image with which you can associate the fact in column A.

Collaborate and Share

In groups of 3 to 5 students, write 1 to 3 questions about the chapter on separate pieces of paper and crumple them into "snowballs," which the instructor collects. The instructor then mixes up the "snowballs" and throws them out to the groups, who then answer and discuss the questions within their group. If you get your own question back, return it to the instructor.

Explain and Learn

Choose a cranial nerve, or the instructor will assign one or more to each class member. Reviewing the information presented in this chapter, as well as in chapters 18-21, gather all the information you can about the cranial nerves to which you were assigned, including their role, how they are assessed, and what range of findings is expected. Class members will present their findings in order, beginning with the first cranial nerve. If more than one student covered the same nerve, go through the order a second or third time.

_____

_____

_____

_____

_____

_____

_____

_____

_____

_____

_____

Relax and Play

1. In small groups, draw a mind map on a piece of poster board, a large piece of butcher paper, or a brown paper grocery bag opened up and spread flat. Draw a circle in the center. In the main circle, place a word or phrase that represents the main point of the chapter. In the secondary or tertiary circles, put words or phrases that represent additional important points. With the members of the group, take turns tossing a coin onto the map. The person tossing the coin explains the term on which the coin landed (or nearest term). Continue until each term is discussed or until instructor calls "time."

2. On a 3" x 5" card, each student writes a question pertaining to the chapter. The cards are collected by the instructor. The instructor, using a koosh ball, small stuffed animal, net bath sponge or some other soft object, asks the question, then tosses the object at random to an individual student who answers the question.

Generalize and Apply

Many eponyms are used in the neurologic examination. Make a list of all the eponymic names appearing in this chapter (such as Hoover sign or Gordon reflex) and jot down a short definition, consulting a medical dictionary as necessary. Keep this list for future reference.

_____

_____

_____

_____

_____

_____

_____

_____

_____

_____

_____

_____

Compare and Contrast

Compare and contrast the *central* and *peripheral* nervous systems. How are they different in structure and function? How are they the same?

_____

_____

_____

_____

Extrapolate and Project

Consider the neurologic examination of a comatose patient described in Short Answer #1. How would the patient's inability to cooperate with the examination interfere with the examination process? What assessments would not be able to be made? What assessments might be modified?

_____

_____

_____

_____

_____

_____

_____

_____

_____

_____

_____

_____

_____

_____

_____

_____

_____

28

The Formal Mental Status Examination

In recording the subject's general appearance at the beginning of the physical examination report, the physician usually comments briefly on mental condition. If the patient displays psychiatric symptoms, the medical examination includes a more formal investigation of mental status. A thorough assessment of a patient's psychiatric condition can take weeks or months, and in a sense is never complete. The mental status examination performed in conjunction with a physical examination is a brief survey of selected aspects of the patient's mental health that can be evaluated without prolonged and intensive interviewing.

Mental status examination demonstrates loose associations, poverty of content of thought, paranoid delusions, and auditory hallucinations.

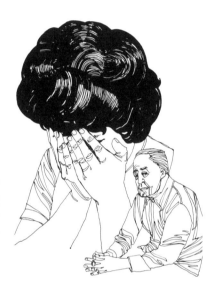

Most of the data for this kind of examination are gathered during history-taking. In addition to the basic historical interview, the examiner asks the subject questions specifically designed to test mental status. The examiner records findings and conclusions according to a fairly standard format. A psychiatrist or other physician with psychiatric leanings may use highly specialized, not to say arcane or extravagant, terminology. The following is a typical format for recording the results of the mental status examination.

Appearance: The examiner records any peculiarities of dress or personal grooming.

neat and well-groomed   carelessly dressed
disheveled, slovenly, unkempt

Sensorium: This refers to the subject's receptiveness and responsiveness to external stimuli. The physician judges alertness, attention span, and ability to receive and process visual, auditory, and tactile stimuli.

alert   short attention span
appears listless and yawns frequently   easily distractable
auditory, finger, tactile, visual agnosia   drowsy, sleepy
delirium   DT's (delirium tremens)
Gerstmann syndrome

Learning Objectives

After careful study of this chapter, you should be able to:

Characterize the mental status exam performed during a routine physical examination.

Classify mental status findings by common format headings.

List findings that describe activity and behavior.

List findings that would indicate a disturbance in thought content.

Explain the phrase "oriented times 3."

Define and discuss the *organic triad*.

Identify formal standardized tests of intelligence and personality.

For Quick Reference

acalculia
acting out
affect
aggression
agoraphobia
ambivalence
amnesia
anhedonia
antalgic gait
apathetic affect
apraxic gait
ataxic gait
attention span
auditory agnosia
auditory hallucinations
auditory stimuli
autistic thinking
automatisms
Bender Gestalt Test
bizarre gestures
blunted affect
BNMSE (Brief Neuropsychological
    Mental Status Examination)
catatonia
catatonic posturing
circumstantial speech
claustrophobia
clumsy gestures
compensation
compulsion
decision-making
déjà vu
delirium
delusions of grandeur
delusions of persecution
depersonalization
depressed affect
disheveled appearance
DT's (delirium tremens)
dysarthric speech
echolalia
echopraxia
egocentricity
ego-defensive mechanisms
ego strength
elated affect
eroticism
euphoric affect
festinating gait
finger agnosia
flat affect
flight of ideas
frustration
Gerstmann syndrome
glue-footed gait
GOAT (Galveston Orientation and
    Amnesia Test)
Goodenough Draw-A-Man Test

Activity and Behavior: Gait, posture, and general level of motor activity are assessed, and any bizarre or compulsive actions, mannerisms, or catatonic posturings are noted.

hyperactive, hyperkinetic	hypoactive, hypokinetic

gait: antalgic, apraxic, ataxic, festinating, glue-footed, hemiplegic, hysterical, propulsion, scissors, shuffling, spastic, steppage, Trendelenburg, waddling, wide-based

gestures: bizarre, clumsy, inappropriate, obscene, purposeless, violent
    fidgeting, picking, handwringing   trichotillomania
catatonia   echopraxia, echolalia   automatisms   *salaam activity*

speech: circumstantial, dysarthric, illogical, inconsequential, halting, *pressured*, rambling, slurred, stuttering, *tangential*

Mood: The subject's emotional state and response to being interviewed are observed and recorded.

affect, mood   Affect is appropriate.
la belle indifférence   calm
agitated, anxious, restless   avoids eye contact, poor eye contact
apathetic, blunted, depressed, elated, euphoric, *flat*, labile, shallow affect
evasive, hostile, suspicious, timid   frank

Thought Content: The physician looks for evidence of unconventional thoughts, fantasies, phobias, hallucinations, delusions, obsessive ideas, or poverty of imagination.

ego   superego   id   ego strength
flight of ideas, loose associations   *word salad*   neologisms
egocentricity   depersonalization
delusion, hallucination, illusion   delusions of grandeur, persecution
obsession, compulsion   ambivalence, conflict, frustration
aggression, hostility   regression   guilt
eroticism   anhedonia
narcissism, autistic thinking   low self-esteem
suicidal ideation
ego-defensive mechanisms   reaction formation
rationalization   acting out   compensation   sublimation
projection   identification   introjection   déjà vu, jamais vu
phobia   rigidity   claustrophobia   agoraphobia

Intellectual Function: The physician tests the speed, coherence, and relevance of the subject's abstract reasoning by posing simple problems in mental arithmetic and asking for interpretations of proverbs such as "Birds of a feather flock together."

acalculia

Orientation: The examiner ascertains the subject's awareness of time (time of day, day of week, date, season, year), place (state, city, exact present location), and person (the subject's own identity and that of family or friends).

oriented times 3 (oriented x 3)

Memory: The subject's recall of recent and remote events is tested through questioning. The examiner also assesses the general fund of information by asking about matters of common knowledge. (Who discovered America?)

amnesia   repression

Judgment: This term refers to the subject's competence or reliability in analyzing facts or situations and deriving conclusions and plans of action from them. (What would you do if you ran out of gas on the interstate?)

decision-making

Insight: In psychiatry, insight means a patient's own awareness of being ill and a recognition of the nature and implications of the illness.

impaired reality testing with denial of illness

Orientation, memory, and judgment are often called the organic triad, because they are commonly affected in organic dementia. In addition to relatively unstructured interviewing, the subject may be given various formal, standardized tests of intelligence and personality.

Halsted-Wepman Aphasia Screening Test

Galveston Orientation and Amnesia Test (GOAT)

Brief Neuropsychological Mental Status Examination (BNMSE)

Stanford-Binet Intelligence Test

Bender Gestalt Test   Rorschach Test

Porteus Maze Test   Minnesota Multiphasic Personality Inventory (MMPI)

For Quick Reference

guilt
hallucination
Halsted-Wepman Aphasia Screening Test
halting speech
handwringing
hemiplegic gait
hostility
hysterical gait
id
identification
illogical speech
illusion
inconsequential speech
insight
intellectual function
intelligence test
introjection
jamais vu
judgment
la belle indifférence
labile affect
listless appearance
loose associations
MMPI (Minnesota Multiphasic Personality Inventory)
mood
narcissism
neat and well-groomed appearance
neologisms
obscene gestures
obsession
organic dementia
organic triad
oriented times 3 (oriented x 3)
paranoid delusions
personality test
phobia
Porteus Maze Test
pressured speech
projection
propulsion gait
purposeless gestures
rambling speech
rationalization
reality testing
recall of recent and remote events
recent and remote memory
regression
repression
Rorschach Test
salaam activity
scissors gait
sentence completion
shallow affect
short attention span
shuffling gait
slovenly appearance

For Quick Reference

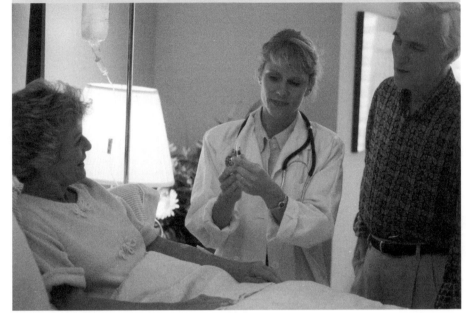

Exercises for Chapter 28

Review and Summarize

A. Multiple Choice

___ 1. The patient's responsiveness to external stimuli is called
   a. Mood.
   b. Orientation.
   c. Sensorium.
   d. Insight.

___ 2. A physician would ask a patient to interpret a proverb such as "A rolling stone gathers no moss" to test
   a. Intellectual function.
   b. Insight.
   c. Judgment.
   d. Memory.

___ 3. A patient who has trouble making decisions and problems analyzing facts or situations is said to have impaired:
   a. Thought content.
   b. Judgment.
   c. Sensorium.
   d. Affect.

B. Fill in the Blank

1. The patient's emotional state and response to being interviewed are recorded as _____.

2. Orientation, memory, and judgment are often called the organic _____.

3. Amnesia and repression are examples of problems with _____.

C. Short Answer

1. To determine if the patient is well oriented, what questions might the examiner ask?

_____

_____

_____

_____

2. Describe the typical format for recording the results of the mental status examination.

_____

_____

_____

_____

3. Write a short definition of the following terms. If you can, condense the definition into just a few words or a single synonym that you feel more comfortable with.

a. Tactile _____

b. Agnosia _____

c. Hemiplegia _____

d. Echolalia _____

e. Automatism _____

f. Dysarthric _____

g. Anhedonia _____

h. Ideation _____

i. Acalculia _____

j. Autism _____

k. Trichotillomania _____

Pause and Reflect

Most of the data for a formal mental status examination are gathered during history-taking. Review the information presented in the categories listed in this chapter and highlight items that are unlikely to have already been obtained earlier in the examination.

Relate and Remember

Draw a mind map to illustrate the 10 typical categories of a formal mental status exam. For each category list the findings, positive or negative, that would be recorded there. Circle the organic triad.

Collaborate and Share

Role-play a formal mental status exam for a patient with schizophrenia. Change roles and choose another diagnosis, such as major depression.

Explain and Learn

In groups of 3 to 5 students, with each group assigned a different section of the chapter, discuss and agree on the important points or main ideas. Put them into your own words. Select one person to present your summary to the class.

Relax and Play

1. Select 10 to 20 words or phrases from the word list in this chapter and create a word search puzzle. Rather than list the words you've chosen, however, list the definitions as clues. Copy the puzzles to share with the rest of the class. Students must first determine which word goes with the definition before finding it in the puzzle.

2. Using the words from the list in the Short Answer questions or at least 10 terms from the word list in the chapter, write a poem or song that incorporates these terms in such a way as to reveal their meaning or use. If writing a song, you can use a familiar tune or rap style.

Generalize and Apply

Write on a 3" x 5" card a statement of something you learned and how you think this information will help you, or a question as yet unanswered. Turn this card in to the instructor as your "ticket out" of class.

Compare and Contrast

What is the difference between a *psychiatrist* and a *psychologist*? Use a medical dictionary or other sources as necessary.

_____

_____

_____

_____

Extrapolate and Project

There are many standardized tests of intelligence and personality, some of which appear in the terms list in this chapter. Where would you find additional information on psychological testing? Compile a list of resources, such as reference books, journals, and Web sites, for future use.

_____

_____

_____

_____

_____

_____

_____

_____

_____

29

The Pediatric History and Physical Examination

The history and physical examination of an infant differ substantially from those of an older child or adult. The entire history must be obtained from sources other than the patient. Parental factors and antenatal events loom large in the history; indeed, a newborn has no other history. The physician must be alert for developmental anomalies and disturbances of nutrition, growth, and maturation that are not diagnostic considerations in later life. On the other hand, degenerative diseases and most kinds of malignancy simply do not occur. Examination techniques are limited to those requiring no cooperation from the patient. Sizes, shapes, textures, and levels of function that would be abnormal in an adult may be perfectly normal in a baby, and vice versa.

> This 6-week-old black infant presents with increasingly severe nonproductive cough, tachypnea, and poor feeding, which developed gradually over the past 4 days.

A newborn undergoes a thorough examination within a few hours after birth. Periodic well-baby checks are part of routine pediatric care. When an infant is admitted to the hospital, a history and physical will be done. Although these examinations vary in scope and emphasis, certain basic points of similarity can be noted. My purpose here is to sketch briefly the pediatric history and physical examination with particular attention to variations from diagnostic procedures used for older children and adults.

The physician precedes the recording of the pediatric history by identifying the informant or informants, their relation to the child, and any emotional or other factors that may affect the accuracy of their information. The chief complaint and history of present illness for a small child are necessarily stated from the viewpoint of the informant.

The past history begins before the child's conception with the health history of the parents and their families and of any older siblings, particularly with respect to hereditary diseases or abnormalities. Pertinent circumstances of the mother's pregnancy include any drug or chemical exposures; use of alcohol, tobacco, or caffeine; exposure to ionizing radiation; maternal infections, particularly rubella or genital herpes; toxemia, hemorrhage, or abnormal weight gain. As full an account as possible is obtained of the labor and delivery, with specific inquiries about gestation time, length of labor, any complications, use of forceps, Apgar score, the child's birth weight, and evidence of congenital anomalies. The child's health during the neonatal period is reviewed, with particular attention to jaundice, respiratory

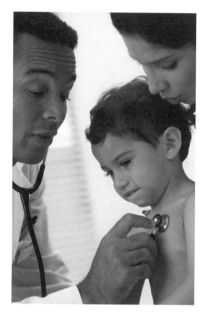

Learning Objectives

After careful study of this chapter, you should be able to:

Explain the ways in which a pediatric H&P differs from that of an adult.

Describe the factors that influence the past history prior to conception.

Give examples of information related to labor and delivery and the neonatal period.

List milestones related to growth and development.

Describe methods of examination unique to the pediatric exam.

Give examples of examination techniques that are modified for a pediatric patient.

Identify tests for reflexes present in normal infants but not in adults.

For Quick Reference

abnormal weight gain
achondroplasia
antenatal events
Apgar score
Barlow sign
Bednar aphthae
body rocking
bottle feeding
brachial palsy
breast feeding
breech baby
bronchiolitis
bulging anterior fontanel
caput succedaneum
cradle cup
cephalopelvic disproportion
cerebral palsy
cesarean section
child abuse
chondrodystrophy
complications of pregnancy
congenital cataract
cranial bosses
craniofacial dysostosis
crepitant rales
cretinism
cri du chat
currant jelly stools
dehydration
DeLange sign
developmental anomalies
diffuse inspiratory crepitant rales
Down syndrome
dysmaturity
encopresis
Erb paralysis (palsy)
erythroblastosis fetalis
exchange transfusion
exstrophy of the bladder
failure to thrive
fecal soiling
feeding difficulties
fontanel
forceps delivery
aftercoming head
Galant reflex
gargoylism
genital herpes
gestation time
grasp reflex
hemorrhage
hereditary diseases
Hurler syndrome
hypotelorism
hypotonic
infantile autism
jaundice
kernicterus

distress, feeding difficulties, fever, or seizures. The nutritional history (breast or bottle feeding, vitamin supplements, weight gain) is reviewed.

Patient was a breech baby delivered at term with forceps to the aftercoming head.
cesarean section at term for cephalopelvic disproportion
Birth weight 8 lb. 10 oz.   Apgar score 7
meconium staining   prolapsed cord
caput succedaneum   prematurity, dysmaturity, postmaturity
Klumpke, Erb paralysis (palsy)   brachial palsy
exstrophy of the bladder   omphalocele
neonatal jaundice, kernicterus   erythroblastosis fetalis
Rh incompatibility   exchange transfusion
respiratory distress   spasmodic croup
breast, bottle feeding   failure to thrive

An important feature of the pediatric history is an account of the child's growth and development. Any available data on height and weight at various ages are collected. Teething history is recorded. Psychomotor development is traced in terms of "milestones" such as acquisition of head control, speech, walking, and toilet training. Social responses and adjustments of the older infant and toddler are evaluated.

currant jelly stools   rice water stools
stooling   encopresis, fecal soiling
infantile autism   toilet training

The physician attempts to learn something of the family's living circumstances (family income, level of intelligence and responsibility of parents, marital harmony and stability, social environment). He is particularly alert for any evidence of child abuse or neglect. In the past medical history, attention is given to routine immunizations against childhood diseases.

child abuse   shaken baby syndrome   sexual abuse   neglect

The examination of a small child calls for much patience and skill. The physician usually solicits the help of a parent or nurse to hold and comfort the child during the examination and to restrain it as needed. Every effort is made to keep the child calm and relaxed because little can be learned by palpating a patient who is writhing or by auscultating one who is screaming.

Down syndrome, mongolism   Hurler syndrome, gargoylism
Morquio syndrome   achondroplasia, chondrodystrophy

Treacher-Collins syndrome   Pierre Robin syndrome

craniofacial dysostosis   ocular hypertelorism, hypotelorism

platybasia   micrognathia

low-set ears   syndactyly

cranial bosses   cretinism

Bednar aphthae   cradle cup

A respiratory rate of 50 breaths a minute.

The child is lethargic and hypotonic with a bulging anterior fontanel.

irritable, cranky   floppy

dehydration   *sunset eyes*

cri du chat

The child's temperature is taken rectally, and blood pressure is determined with a suitably sized cuff. Height (length) and weight are recorded, as well as the circumferences of the head and the chest. Throughout the examination the physician is particularly alert for evidence of congenital or developmental abnormalities. The skin is evaluated for jaundice, rashes, or signs of dehydration. Any deformity or abnormal enlargement of the head is noted, and the fontanels are palpated. The eyes are examined for strabismus, congenital cataract, and signs of infection. Vision can be tested in preschool children with a eye chart consisting entirely of E's printed in various positions. The child uses three fingers to show which way the crosspieces of each E are pointing.

Examination of ears, nose, and throat is often a trying experience for both examiner and subject. Assistance is essential. Auscultation of the lungs of a crying child may have to be confined to the inspiratory phase of respiration. The heart is examined for evidence of congenital anomalies. Palpation of the abdomen is performed carefully to detect malignant tumors, which occasionally occur in quite small children, and umbilical or inguinal hernias. Examination of the genitalia and rectum is generally limited to external inspection unless disease or injury of these structures is suspected.

short, tight frenulum   diffuse inspiratory crepitant rales

bronchiolitis   Wilms tumor

mild subcostal retractions

In the orthopedic examination, the physician looks for evidence of congenital malformations or injuries, and pays particular attention to the hip joints, legs, and feet. The neurologic examination of a small child includes tests for reflexes that are present in normal infants but not in older children or adults. These include the Moro (startle), grasp, rooting, and tonic neck reflexes. Alertness, muscle tone, and general responsiveness to stimuli are assessed with due consideration of the child's age.

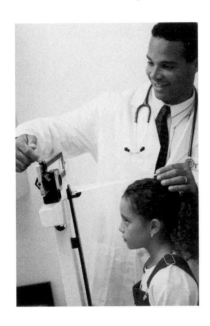

Barlow sign   rockerbottom foot
Ortolani sign, test   spastic diplegia
telescoping hip   cerebral palsy
Moro reflex   tonic neck reflex   grasp reflex   righting reflex
rooting reflex   body rocking   DeLange sign   Landau reflex
Galant reflex

Exercises for Chapter 29

Review and Summarize

A. Multiple Choice

____ 1. The pediatric patient's history begins
   a. Before conception.
   b. Just after conception.
   c. The first time the mother feels the fetus move (quickening).
   d. Just before birth.
   e. Just after birth.

____ 2. What eye chart is most often used for children?
   a. M.
   b. Snellen.
   c. E.
   d. Jaeger.
   e. Both C and D.

B. Fill in the Blank

1. A child's psychomotor development, such as speaking, and walking, is traced in terms of

   _____ .

2. Enlargement of the _____ is often gauged by circumferential measurement and

   palpation of the fontanels.

C. Short Answer

1. What problems during the neonatal period are given particular attention on history-taking?

   _____

   _____

2. List the reflexes that are normally present in babies and small children but not in adults.

   _____

   _____

3. Write a short definition of the following terms. If you can, condense the definition into just a few words or a single synonym that you feel more comfortable with.

a. Fontanel _____

b. Boss _____

c. Frenulum _____

d. Croup _____

e. Meconium _____

f. Omphalocele _____

g. Syndactyly _____

h. Cretinism _____

i. Diplegia _____

j. Gestation _____

k. Cri du chat _____

Pause and Reflect

Using different colored highlighters or crayons, underline or highlight important points or main ideas of the chapter. Circle key words. Use symbols meaningful to you (such as stars, asterisks, exclamation point, question mark, etc.) to mark key words and phrases. Summarize the information you thought most important from the chapter. If you had any questions, write those out to share with classmates or to ask your instructor.

_____

_____

_____

_____

_____

_____

_____

Relate and Remember

Using this outline of the human body, list 3 to 5 terms for each area that the physician might use to describe the findings in that area.

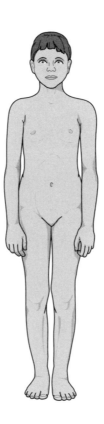

Collaborate and Share

Label a blank sheet of paper with your name at the top and write a question requiring a short answer (less than a sentence) related to this chapter. Pass this paper to the student on your right, who will answer the question and then add a question of his or her own, as you answer the question on the paper received from the student on your left. Each sheet moves around the room until everyone has had a turn with every paper and you end up with the paper with your name at the top. Choose the best question(s) and answer(s) from your page to read aloud when called upon by your instructor.

Explain and Learn

List everything you know about this chapter. As a group, pick 1 to 3 most important points and share with the class.

_____

_____

_____

_____

_____

_____

_____

_____

_____

_____

_____

_____

_____

Relax and Play

1. In small groups, role-play the routine history and physical examination of a 6-year-old. One student will act as patient, another as parent, and another as the examining physician.

2. After reviewing the chapter as a class or in small groups, the instructor will announce "Go," and individual class members will "pop up" and call out one important fact learned, already known, or remembered about a topic or section in this chapter. If a student answers correctly, the instructor tosses the student a "fun size" candy bar.

Generalize and Apply

Type on a separate sheet or handwrite below a complete history and physical examination for a fictitious pediatric patient. Record all the historical information described in the chapter, including both positive and negative findings.

_____

_____

_____

_____

_____

_____

_____

_____

_____

_____

_____

Compare and Contrast

How is the physical examination of a pediatric patient different from that of an adult? How are they similar?

_____

_____

_____

_____

_____

_____

_____

Extrapolate and Project

Research a congenital anomaly of your choice or assigned by your instructor. Prepare a 1-2 page report or a 10-minute oral presentation to share your findings, or summarize your findings below.

_____

_____

_____

_____

_____

_____

_____

_____

_____

_____

_____

_____

_____

30

Diagnostic Formulations

The performance of a history and physical examination is not a mere ritual, however much it may seem so at times to both physician and patient. The purpose, product, or "bottom line" of diagnostic assessment is a diagnosis. The formulation of a diagnosis is the pivotal point in the doctor-patient interaction where investigation culminates and gives way to intervention. As described in the Introduction, diagnosis in this context usually means the name of a disease. The label assigned may be more or less precise (and correct) depending on the success of the diagnostic effort: *varicella* as opposed to *acute febrile exanthem; gastroesophageal reflux disease with peptic esophagitis* as opposed to *chest pain, cause undetermined.*

Dx (diagnosis)

When, as often happens, the history and physical examination are recorded before x-rays, laboratory tests, and other special procedures have supplied data for a firm and narrow diagnostic label, the physician may conclude the history and physical examination report with a *tentative (provisional, working) diagnosis*. For a patient just admitted to the hospital, this translates to *admitting diagnosis*. The physician's phrase *rule out*, as in "rule out myocardial infarction," is sometimes misunderstood. This expression does not mean that the diagnosis has been ruled out, but rather that, although less than probable, it remains enough of a possibility to require further consideration. When such a possibility is confirmed after all, it is said, somewhat quaintly, to have been *ruled in*. At the conclusion of the diagnostic process a final diagnosis is recorded. In a hospital record this is called a *discharge diagnosis* (assuming that the patient leaves the hospital alive). In surgical cases, preoperative and postoperative diagnoses are recorded.

admitting, preoperative, provisional, tentative, working diagnosis

discharge, final, postmortem, postoperative diagnosis

The choice of diagnostic language is presently governed by many factors extraneous to the purely practical question of a basis or starting point for treatment. Virtually all health insurance companies and other third-party payers of medical expenses require healthcare providers to use standard disease nomenclature in filing claims, and gear specific dollar limits on payments to specific diagnostic categories. Hence any physician, clinic, hospital, clinical laboratory, or

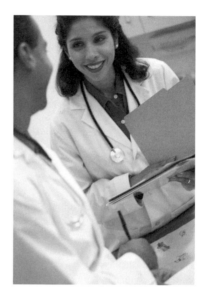

Learning Objectives

After careful study of this chapter, you should be able to:

Compare and contrast provisional and final diagnoses.

Explain why the phrase *rule out* is often misunderstood.

Justify the need for a common diagnostic language.

Differentiate between the two primary sources for official nomenclature.

Discuss and give examples of diagnostic labels that are changed due to associated unfavorable connotations.

Employ qualifying adjectives, etiologic terms, and staging formats in a diagnosis.

Identify terminology associated with diagnostic formulations.

For Quick Reference

pharmacy that expects to be paid for services rendered must speak the same diagnostic language as the prospective payer.

In the United States, the generally accepted official nomenclature is the *International Classification of Diseases* (ICD), prepared and published under the auspices of the World Health Organization and revised annually. Besides being extremely well organized, the ICD has the advantage of providing a number code for each diagnosis. Numerical coding streamlines many aspects of health information management; however, consistently accurate coding requires considerable training and experience. In addition to diagnoses, medical services are numerically coded; in this country the standard is *Current Procedural Terminology* (CPT), published by the American Medical Association.

Diagnostic labels are used by various committees and agencies for purposes of classification and analysis. Peer-review committees assessing the degree to which individual physicians follow professional standards key their investigations to specific admitting and discharge diagnoses in hospital charts. Hospital administrators, credentialing bodies, and public agencies compile statistics on the basis of recorded diagnoses.

Certain well-established diagnostic labels with unfavorable connotations have recently been supplanted by others considered less objectionable. Thus *drug addiction* becomes *chemical dependence*; *mongolism*, *Down syndrome*. *Fibrocystic disease of the breast* has been renamed *fibrocystic condition of the breast* for at least two reasons. Life insurance companies have seized upon the homely and harmless word *disease* as a reason to deny coverage or to increase premiums, and patients themselves seem much less alarmed by having a *condition* than a *disease*. Similarly, physicians continue to seek less threatening synonyms for terms such as *arthritis*, *tumor*, and *functional heart murmur*.

To labels that specify particular injuries, diseases, or abnormalities (*incised wound, myocardial infarction, sigmoid diverticulosis*), physicians append many qualifying adjectives to indicate whether they are local or general, acute or chronic, constant or intermittent, symptomatic or asymptomatic, early or late in their course, typical or atypical. Etiologic terms are also added, particularly terms that distinguish primary from secondary conditions and organic from functional ones. It may be important to indicate that a condition is a complication or sequela of another condition.

focal hemorrhage, localized eruption, regional enteritis

diffuse fibrosing interstitial lung disease, disseminated intravascular coagulation, generalized arteriosclerosis, multiple sclerosis, systemic candidiasis

acute myocardial infarction, chronic bronchitis, subacute thyroiditis

Hodgkin disease in remission, stroke in progress

dormant herpes simplex, early diabetes mellitus, end-stage renal failure, late benign syphilis, latent schizophrenia, prodromal roseola, tardive dyskinesia, terminal leukemia

hereditary spherocytosis, acquired immunodeficiency syndrome

infantile autism, juvenile rheumatoid arthritis, presenile dementia, senile vaginitis

fatal, lethal, life-threatening

endemic goiter, epidemic conjunctivitis

dysfunctional uterine bleeding, functional bowel syndrome, organic brain syndrome

etiology undetermined   FUO (fever of undetermined origin)

agnogenic myeloid metaplasia, endogenous depression, essential dysmenorrhea, idiopathic thrombocytopenic purpura, primary hyperparathyroidism, spontaneous pneumothorax

exogenous obesity, secondary hypertension, iatrogenic hypokalemia, dermatitis medicamentosa

asymptomatic bacteriuria, occult malignancy, silent myocardial infarction, subclinical giardiasis, impending hepatic coma

florid cirrhosis, frank hemorrhage, fulminant hepatitis, massive embolism

intractable pain, refractory asthma, insulin-resistant diabetes mellitus

status epilepticus, hypertensive crisis

complications, residuals, *sequelae*   complex, syndrome, tetralogy, triad

Scabies should probably be included in the differential (diagnosis).

documented episode   factitial, factitious

protean   pathognomonic   malingering   Munchausen syndrome

Various types of classification or quantification may be combined with diagnoses. A prognosis is a prediction of the outcome of the disease. For many diseases, stages have been established according to standard criteria. A common staging format for malignancies is the TNM (tumor-node-metastasis) classification. For example, T2a, N1b, M0 for a breast cancer means "primary tumor between 2 and 5 cm in size, with no fixation to underlying pectoral fascia or muscle; movable axillary nodes on the same side, believed to contain cancer; no distant metastases known." The degree of disability arising from an illness or injury may be estimated in qualitative or quantitative terms as part of a diagnostic formulation. Such an estimate can have a bearing on the patient's employability or on compensation or disability payments.

prognosis: excellent, favorable, good, grave, guarded, poor, unfavorable

benign, malignant   metastatic

Apgar score   Glasgow coma level

New York Heart Association functional class III

PULSES (**p**hysical condition, **u**pper extremity function, **l**ower extremity function, **s**ensory and communication abilities, **e**xcretory control, **s**ocial support)

For Quick Reference

infantile autism
insulin-resistant diabetes mellitus
International Classification of Diseases (ICD)
intractable pain
juvenile rheumatoid arthritis
late benign syphilis
latent schizophrenia
lethal
life-threatening
localized eruption
malingering
massive embolism
metastatic
mongolism
multiple sclerosis
Munchausen syndrome
myocardial infarction
occult malignancy
organic brain syndrome
pathognomonic
peptic esophagitis
poor prognosis
postmortem diagnosis
postoperative
preoperative
presenile dementia
primary hyperparathyroidism
prodromal roseola
prognosis
protean
provisional diagnosis
PULSES
refractory asthma
regional enteritis
residuals
scabies
secondary hypertension
senile vaginitis
sequelae
sigmoid diverticulosis
silent myocardial infarction
spontaneous pneumothorax
standard disease nomenclature
status epilepticus
stroke in progress
subacute thyroiditis
subclinical giardiasis
systemic candidiasis
tardive dyskinesia
tentative diagnosis
terminal leukemia
tetralogy
TNM (tumor-node-metastasis) classification
triad
unfavorable prognosis
working diagnosis

Exercises for Chapter 30

Review and Summarize

A. Multiple Choice

___ 1. For purposes of classification and analysis, the World Health Organization publishes a list of diseases with number codes assigned to each. This publication is the
   a. *Physicians' Desk Reference.*
   b. *International Classification of Diseases.*
   c. *Current Procedural Terminology.*
   d. *WHO Global Guide to Diagnosis and Procedure.*

___ 2. Physician peer-review committees who evaluate the work of other physicians depend largely on
   a. The physician's reputation.
   b. Departmental statistics.
   c. Grand rounds and noon conferences.
   d. The patient's medical chart.

___ 3. A common classification for malignant tumors is
   a. MTC.
   b. ABC.
   c. 1-2-3.
   d. TNM.

B. Fill in the Blank

1. The bottom line of diagnostic assessment (history and physical, laboratory tests, imaging studies) is to reach a

   tentative or working _____.

2. A _____ is the prediction of the outcome of a disease.

C. Short Answer

1. Explain the phrase "rule out."

   _____

   _____

   _____

   _____

2. Why is standard disease nomenclature required by health insurance companies?

_____

_____

_____

_____

3. Why are numerical codes used to report medical conditions and treatment?

_____

_____

_____

_____

4. Write a short definition of the following terms. If you can, condense the definition into just a few words or a single synonym that you feel more comfortable with.

a. Postmortem _____

b. Nomenclature _____

c. Sequela _____

d. Disseminated_____

e. Subacute _____

f. Endogenous _____

g. Fulminant _____

h. Embolism _____

i. Tetralogy _____

j. Malingering _____

k. Protean _____

l. Metastasis _____

Pause and Reflect

Read this chapter aloud, by yourself or taking turns with other students. If you don't know the meaning or pronunciation of a word, you should look it up. As you read, pause and reflect on key points at the end of each section. Make notes in the margins of your book, mark with dots or stars, and draw lines from key ideas to subordinate points. Summarize your reading in outline form below.

_____

_____

_____

_____

_____

_____

_____

_____

_____

_____

_____

Relate and Remember

Take a sheet of paper and draw lines to create four columns, labeled A through D. List five important things to remember about the chapter. Put these in column A. In column B, next to each of the items to remember, write the name of an object that might help you to remember the fact. In column C, write the name of a place that might help you to remember the fact. In column D, write a description of a visual image with which you can associate the fact in column A.

Collaborate and Share

After you have read the chapter, form groups of 3 to 5. Divide the chapter so that each group has a portion. Reread your section. As a group, write questions based on your section. They may be multiple choice, short answer, or fill in the blank. The number of questions will depend on how large a section of the chapter your group is covering. Pass your questions to the next group, working clockwise around the room, until every group has had the opportunity to answer all the questions.

Explain and Learn

Individually, using colored dots (or a drawn dot or star), mark what you feel is the most important point or line in each paragraph. If you feel there are multiple important points, rate them and mark the most important with, for example, a red dot, a secondary point with a yellow dot, and the least important point with a green dot. Once you have done this, share your findings with two or three classmates near you. Do you all agree? Discuss any differences of opinion and justify your final decisions. Outline your findings below.

_____

_____

_____

_____

_____

_____

_____

_____

_____

_____

_____

Relax and Play

1. Fold a blank piece of paper in half three times so that when unfolded there are eight squares. Write one thing you learned in each square. Move around the room, asking other students to define or explain an item on your sheet. That student then signs the square. The student who gets all eight squares signed first wins.

2. On a 3" x 5" card, each student writes a question pertaining to the chapter. The cards are collected by the instructor. The instructor, using a koosh ball, small stuffed animal, net bath sponge or some other soft object, asks the question, then tosses the object at random to an individual student who answers the question.

Generalize and Apply

Choose 10 diseases from the list of terms accompanying this chapter. For each disease, draw a small mind map with the name of the disease in the center. In surrounding circles add three to five adjectives that could apply to this disease from the list that appears in the paragraph that begins, "To labels that specify particular injuries." Include qualifying adjectives, etiologic terms, and any classifications or quantification as appropriate.

Compare and Contrast

Diagnoses and medical services are numerically coded using the standards set forth in the *International Classification of Disease* (ICD) and *Current Procedural Terminology* (CPT). How are these publications similar and how do they differ? If possible, examine these texts first hand and describe the differences in the way information is arranged. Describe how you would look something up in each text. If you don't have them available in your classroom or school library, try a public library or the medical library of a hospital in your community.

_____

_____

_____

_____

_____

Extrapolate and Project

Diagnostic labels with unfavorable connotations are sometimes changed to less objectionable ones: *Down syndrome* instead of *mongolism condition* instead of *disease*. Discuss the reasons for this trend. Can you think of situations where adopting a less threatening term might ultimately have a negative impact on patient care or the health care system in general? Propose new names for diagnostic labels that you find objectionable.

Glossary

ab (AB). Abortion or miscarriage. *AB2*: The patient has had 2 abortions or miscarriages.

acute abdomen. An abdomen showing signs of acute inflammation.

adnexa (singular, *adnexum*). The uterine appendages, including the ovary and tube on each side. Adnexa is plural: "The adnexa were unremarkable."

air hunger. Extreme dyspnea, with gasping and other evidence of respiratory distress.

air-bone gap. In the Rinne test (see Chap. 20), the persistence of hearing by bone conduction after hearing by air conduction has ceased.

alar flaring. Flaring (dilatation) of the nostrils on inspiration, sometimes the only sign of dyspnea in a small child.

allergic salute. An unconscious maneuver often repeated by children with allergic rhinitis to improve air flow through nostrils blocked by congestion. It consists of pressing up and back on the tip of the nose, usually with the heel of the hand.

allergic shiners. Darkening of the skin around the eyes, resembling periorbital hematomas, as a symptom of allergic rhinitis.

apron. Excessive subcutaneous fat that hangs from the abdominal wall like an apron.

bark (verb). To abrade the skin.

benign. Not malignant. Not diseased. Normal, not showing evidence of disease or abnormality.

bishop's nod. Rhythmic nodding of the head, synchronous with the pulse, in aortic regurgitation.

bite line. A horizontal line of whitened, thickened buccal mucosa caused by habitual biting or chewing of the surface.

black hairy tongue. Discoloration and alteration of the surface texture of the tongue by fungal infection.

blackout (lay term). Syncope; loss of consciousness.

bleed. A hemorrhage, usually gastrointestinal.

blown pupil. A dilated and fixed pupil.

blue bloater. A patient with severe respiratory failure showing dyspnea, cyanosis, and peripheral edema due to right ventricular failure.

boxcarring. Segmentation of blood in retinal vessels; a sign of death.

bouche de tapir. Elongation of the face, so that it resembles that of a tapir, caused by extreme weakness of the muscles about the mouth.

buffalo hump. A zone of focal edema over the upper and midback, seen especially in Cushing syndrome and after prolonged adrenal corticosteroid therapy.

bull's eye lesion. A skin lesion with concentric rings, resembling a target.

butterflies in the stomach (lay term). A sensation of nausea or uneasiness in the upper abdomen, often due to anxiety.

butterfly rash. A rash of the malar eminences that has a shape roughly like that of a butterfly.

canker sore (lay term). Aphtha; aphthous ulcer.

carphologia. Purposeless plucking at clothing or bedclothes; sometimes seen in dementia or terminal illness.

catch (lay term). A sharp, localized pain, usually in the chest and provoked or aggravated by inspiration.

cauliflower ear (lay term). An external ear deformed by repeated or severe trauma, as in boxers and wrestlers.

chandelier sign. Extreme tenderness of the uterine adnexa, elicited on pelvic examination. (The term fancifully implies that the pain causes the patient to leap into the air and cling to the chandelier.)

Charley horse (lay term). Painful spasm in a lower extremity, generally due to injury.

chart. The entire record of a patient's hospitalization.

checking. Fine control of voluntary movement; the act of stopping a motion when its goal or purpose has been attained.

choke, choked disk. Edema of the optic nerve head, as seen on funduscopic examination.

Christmas-tree pattern. Distribution of cutaneous lesions on the back characteristic of pityriasis rosea.

chronic. Persistent or prolonged, as in chronic bronchitis, chronic steroid therapy.

clap (lay term). Gonorrhea.

cobblestoning. Coarsely lumpy appearance of a mucosal surface, such as the tongue or conjunctiva, caused by inflammation.

cogwheel breathing. Jerkiness or intermittency of breath sounds on inspiration, due to sudden expansion of previously collapsed air sacs.

compensated. Corrected or mitigated; said of a defect or disability, as, *compensated hearing loss*, hearing loss improved with a hearing aid; *edentulous and compensated*, toothless but fitted with dentures.

compliance. A patient's following of a physician's directions and advice regarding diet or medicinal treatment.

compromise. Impairment or damage to a normal structure or function, as in neural compromise, circulatory compromise.

copper wire effect. Narrowing of arterioles in the retina.

cracked-pot note. The sound elicited by percussing the skull in hydrocephalus.

cramps (lay term). Dysmenorrhea.

cri du chat (French, "cat's cry"). A high-pitched whining cry noted in brain-injured children and in newborns with cri du chat syndrome, which includes deformity and mental retardation.

crick (lay term). Painful spasm, usually in the neck.

DES daughter. A girl or woman exposed in utero to diethylstilbestrol (DES), formerly prescribed for bleeding and other complications of pregnancy and now known to affect fetal development of the genital tract.

dewlap. Redundant skin hanging below the chin.

diamond-shaped murmur. A systolic heart murmur that first grows louder and then grows softer. The term alludes to its appearance on a phonocardiogram.

documented. Proved by objective diagnostic tests or examinations.

dowager's hump. Kyphosis due to osteoporosis of the spine.

downgoing. Said of the normal response to the Babinski test, in which the great toe curls downward when the sole of the foot is stroked.

dry heaves. Gagging or retching without emesis.

duck waddle. A test of the integrity of the knee joints and menisci, in which the patient is required to "walk" in a squatting position.

empty nest syndrome. Restlessness and depression in a woman whose children have grown up and left home.

engaged, engagement. Said of the fetal head as it enters and becomes lodged in the superior pelvic strait.

episode. An attack or incident of illness.

ethanolism. Alcoholism.

exquisite(ly). Said of extremely severe pain or tenderness.

fabere. An acronym for the maneuvers of the Patrick test for hip joint disease: flexion, abduction, external rotation, and extension.

fadir. An acronym for maneuvers used to test the hip joint: flexion, adduction, and internal rotation.

falling out (lay term). Syncope; loss of consciousness.

fester (lay term). Suppurate.

fetal small parts. The extremities of a fetus as felt through the mother's abdominal wall.

flat(tened) affect. Diminished emotional response; apathy.

flooding (lay term). Very heavy menstrual flow.

follow. To provide continuing supervision or care of a patient's medical condition.

foot drop. Passive plantar flexion of the foot due to paralysis of dorsiflexor muscles.

fortification spectrum. A jagged formation of bright lines sometimes experienced by the patient as an aura of migraine headache and in other conditions.

friable. Crumbly; easily broken up or damaged.

frog in the throat (lay term). Hoarseness.

fungus (lay term). Used generically of many skin conditions, and also of otitis externa.

galling. Chafing of apposed skin surfaces, as in the groin; intertrigo.

game (lay term). Impaired by injury or disease; usually applied to the lower extremity.

gathering (lay term). Suppuration.

geographic tongue. A condition of the tongue in which irregular zones of redness appear and create an appearance somewhat like a map.

gimpy (lay term). Said of a lower extremity in which pain, spasm, or deformity causes a limp.

globus hystericus. The sensation of a lump in the throat, sometimes accompanied by choking, due to emotional upset.

glue-footed gait. An ataxic gait in which the patient seems unable to lift either foot from the floor.

goose-egg (lay term). Traumatic hematoma of the scalp.

gravida (G). Pregnant. In medical jargon, the number of pregnancies a woman has had; *Gravida 4* (G4): having been pregnant 4 times.

haircut (lay term). Syphilitic chancre.

hot potato voice. A hollow voice caused by edema or paralysis of the soft palate; most commonly observed in severe pharyngitis or peritonsillar abscess.

hypnotic. A drug used to induce sleep.

intact. Structurally and functionally unaffected by injury or disease.

in extremis. At the point of death.

intoeing. Turning in of the forefoot in walking.

I:E ratio. Inspiratory:expiratory ratio, the ratio between the duration of inspiration and that of expiration. (Dictated as "I to E ratio.")

jacksonian march. Progression of a jacksonian seizure from one muscle group to adjacent areas or to a generalized motor seizure.

joint mice. Loose fragments of cartilage or other material within the synovial capsule of a joint.

lancinating. Stabbing, piercing (of a pain).

lid lag. Abnormally sluggish movement of the upper eyelid over the eye in exophthalmos.

lie. The relative position of the long axis of a fetus with respect to that of the mother: longitudinal or transverse.

liver flap. Asterixis; a coarse flapping tremor of the hands, so called because it is often seen in hepatic failure.

logorrhea. Extreme loquacity; a copious flow of talk, often incoherent.

macular fan, macular star. A fan- or star-shaped folding or pleating of the retina due to edema.

maintain. To control or limit the effects of an illness or abnormal state with diet, medicine, or other means.

moon face. Pronounced rounding of the cheeks in Cushing syndrome or prolonged adrenocortical therapy.

moribund. Dying.

morsicatio buccarum. The nervous habit of biting or chewing the buccal mucosa.

overshooting. Failure to stop a voluntary movement when its goal or purpose has been achieved.

para (P). Denotes the number of times a woman has delivered a child. *Para 3* (P3): having had 3 deliveries.

parity. A woman's reproductive history.

pathognomonic. Characteristic or diagnostic of a particular disease.

pathology. In medical jargon, denotes any disease or abnormality.

peau d'orange (French, "orange peel"). A dimpled appearance of the skin due to interstitial edema and seen particularly in breast cancer.

pill-rolling tremor. Involuntary rhythmic opposing movements of the thumb and fingers, characteristic of parkinsonism.

pink puffer. A patient with early respiratory failure, showing dyspnea but no cyanosis.

pinkeye (lay term). Any condition causing hyperemia of one or both eyes; usually, bacterial or viral conjunctivitis.

pipestem sheathing. An appearance created by lipid deposition along retinal arterioles.

post-tussive. After coughing. Applied to rales and rhonchi that do not disappear after the patient tries to clear the trachea and bronchi by coughing.

present (verb). To present oneself to a physician, clinic, or hospital for treatment.

presentation. (1) The initial overt features of an illness. (2) The part of a fetus that enters the birth canal first; also, presenting part.

pressured speech. A rapid, tense manner of speaking that betrays the anxiety of the speaker.

proprietary (medicine). Nonprescription medicine.

protean. Said of a disease having various symptoms in different patients.

pulse deficit. The arithmetical difference between the apical pulse and the radial or other peripheral pulse. Generally it indicates the number of cardiac contractions per minute that are not sufficiently strong to generate a peripheral pulse.

rabbit nose. Habitual repeated wrinkling of the nose by a person with itching of the nares due to allergic rhinitis.

rabbit stools. Stools expelled as small lumps.

raccoon eye(s). Discoloration below or around the eye(s) due to subcutaneous hemorrhage, sometimes seen in basal skull fracture.

residual(s). Lasting effects of disease or injury.

ribbon stools. Stools of greatly diminished caliber, often due to partial obstruction of the lower bowel by a tumor.

root signs. Signs of compression or injury of spinal nerve roots, such as absence of deep tendon reflexes in a patient with a herniated intervertebral disk.

running. Producing abnormal or excessive secretions.

salaam activity. Involuntary gestures of head and arms resembling the salute given in Eastern countries, observed in psychomotor epilepsy and other neurologic disorders.

sand (lay term). Inspissated secretions in or about the eyes.

scrim. Slang for auditory discrimination.

sentinel node. An enlarged lymph node in the left supraclavicular fossa containing cancer metastatic from the stomach, also called Virchow or Troisier node; more generally, any palpable lymph node indicating malignancy.

sentinel pile. A hemorrhoid or hemorrhoidlike nodule of tissue that forms below an anal fissure.

sequela (usually used in plural, *sequelae*). A persistent effect of an illness or injury, such as paralysis after a stroke.

shin splints (lay term). Painful spasm of shin muscles due to strain, usually as a result of running.

shiner (lay term). Periorbital ecchymosis.

shocky. In shock, or showing signs (tachycardia, pallor, diaphoresis, restlessness) suggestive of shock.

significant other. One bound by intimate personal ties to another; usually a lover.

silent. Without symptoms or signs, as in silent gallstones, silent myocardial infarction.

silver wire effect. An effect created by narrowing of arterioles in the retina.

sleep (lay term). Inspissated mucus in the eyes.

smarting (lay term). Pain, usually of a stinging or burning character, particularly in the eye.

spiking fever. A fever characterized by recurrent sudden brief elevations, which look like a row of spikes on a temperature graph.

splinter hemorrhage. A short linear hemorrhage under a fingernail or toenail, longitudinally oriented and looking somewhat like a splinter; often due to trauma but sometimes a sign of infective endocarditis.

spotting. Scanty vaginal bleeding, menstrual or otherwise.

star figure. A star-shaped folding or pleating of the retina due to edema.

status post. The condition or fact of having sustained an injury or illness or having undergone a surgical procedure, as in *status post appendectomy*.

stepping of vessels. Abrupt change in the direction of retinal vessels passing over the brim of an abnormally deep optic cup.

steroid. Adrenocortical steroid.

stitch (lay term). A sharp, localized pain in the chest wall, often provoked or aggravated by respiratory movements.

stooling. Defecation; used generally of infants not yet toilet-trained.

stoved (lay term). Of an extremity, stubbed; injured by direct concussion.

sundowning. Increase in confusion, delirium, or agitation after dark, common in senile and other dementias.

sunset eyes. An abnormal appearance of the eyes in which the pupils lie at or below the level of the lower lids; seen in infantile hydrocephalus and due to retraction of the upper lids.

surgical. Referring to a condition that requires surgical treatment, as in surgical abdomen.

tangential speech. Rambling, tending to go off on tangents.

taper. To reduce the dose of a medicine gradually.

target lesion. A skin lesion consisting of concentric rings of erythema.

tic. (1) Slang for diverticulum. (2) An involuntary repetitive movement.

titrate. To make fine adjustments in the dose of a medicine by observing its effects.

toeing in, out. Turning the forefoot in or out in walking.

toileting. Using bathroom facilities without assistance; said in connection with partially disabled persons.

toxic. Showing signs of toxemia or septicemia, such as fever, tachycardia, flushing, and mental confusion.

tracheal tug. A downward impulse imparted to the trachea by an aortic aneurysm, synchronous with heartbeat.

trigger point. A localized zone of tenderness, especially in a muscle.

uncompensated. See *compensated*.

upgoing. Describing the movement of the great toe in the Babinski reflex.

ventilate. To express verbally, especially as a release for pent-up emotions.

verbalize. To formulate in words; often simply jargon for "talk."

water brash. Regurgitation of excessive saliva from the esophagus, often combined with some gastric juice.

wean. To discontinue a medicine by gradually reducing the dose.

weal, welp, welt (lay terms). Wheal, papule.

wen. A sebaceous cyst or other bland swelling on, in, or under the skin.

whelp (lay term). Wheal, papule.

word salad. Incoherent speech, as sometimes observed in schizophrenia or stroke patients.

work up. To perform a thorough diagnostic evaluation or *workup*.

wrist drop. Passive flexion of the wrist due to paralysis of extensor muscles.

zit (lay term). Comedo; acne pustule.

Answers to Exercises

Note: Answers to objective questions are provided, including sample responses to selected questions requiring a narrative response. Refer to **About the Exercises** (page vi) for additional information.

Introduction

A. Multiple choice
1. C
2. B
3. D
4. B

B. Fill in the Blank
1. abstraction
2. nosology
3. provisional
4. anamnesis
5. physical (examination)

C. Short Answer
1. individual; personal; as perceived by patient
2. impartial; based on observation
3. abnormalities in tissue, structure, or processes caused by disease
4. names
5. practical; observed; not theoretical
6. conclusion; deduction
7. misleading information
8. complex; obscure
9. obscure; esoteric
10. A skillfully obtained history supplies both a larger number of diagnostic clues and more useful and specific ones than the physical examination. It is the summary of the patient's symptoms and the course of the illness. The physical examination is the objective observance of the signs of disease. It does not involve elaborate diagnostic procedures that require specialized instruments or machines. The H&P will contain more negatives than positives because the physician is not concerned merely with a list of abnormalities but the complete picture of a patient's condition, which includes the common or relevant signs and symptoms that are not present. The language of an H&P may be formal, informal, institutional, regional, or individual and may not appear in conventional references. It is economic, abbreviated, condensed, lacking complete sentences and strict grammatical structure. The language may be obscure, esoteric, abstract, or technical rather than plain and simple.

Explain and Learn
1. Disease is a unifying concept by which physicians attempt to explain the origin and interrelations of symptoms and malfunctions and an attempt to simplify and streamline their thinking about illness. Every disease is expressed differently in each individual, but there are enough similarities that symptoms can be classified and categorized as a disease or syndrome.
2. The history provides a larger number of more useful and more specific clues to the diagnosis than does the physical exam.

Extrapolate and Project
1. (There are multiple solutions to this question and it is anticipated that each student will produce a unique visual interpretation.)
2. Studying the text will help me understand the structure of the history and physical examination. It will also introduce me to a large body of terminology specific to the history and physical.

Chapter 1

A. Multiple Choice
1. D
2. A

B. Fill in the Blank
1. written records and/or someone else
2. scope

C. Short Answer
1. Factors include the informant's memory and intelligence, ability and willingness to communicate, anxiety, lack of knowledge or misunderstanding of medicine or body function, deliberate false or misleading information, and how questions are worded.
2. a. stubbornly; resolutely
   b. claims; asserts
   c. irrelevant; unrelated
   d. wordiness; talkativeness
   e. unconsciously turns fact into fantasy; lies
   f. uncontrollably repeats
   g. lying; false
   h. demarcated; established by border or boundary
   i. subtly or stealthily spreading
   j. undiminished; not decreased
   k. undiminished; not decreased
   l. shifting; changing; alternating
   m. fierce; intense
   n. alleviated; mollified
   o. provoking; stimulating

Relate and Remember
Sample response: It is like a ball of twine because each layer of string represents a piece of information. A knot in the string might be an incorrect piece of information caused by the patient's inability to communicate or deliberate fabrication. The entire ball of

string represents the sum total of all the information obtained from the patient.

Chapter 2

A. Multiple Choice
1. C
2. A

B. Fill in the Blank
1. chief complaint (CC); history of present illness (HPI)
2. history of present illness (HPI)
3. chronologic
4. duration

C. Short Answer
1. It contains all the details leading up to and/or pertaining to the patient's current complaint.
2. Onset of symptoms may be subtle and unrecognized; unrelated symptoms may occur together.
3. a. in a cursory or superficial manner
   b. main; primary; chief
   c. occurring prior to onset of present complaint
   d. condition making one susceptible to an illness
   e. aggravate; worsen
   f. minor ailment
   g. weakness; debility
   h. listlessness
   i. infirmity; weakness
   j. as relates to medicine; a brand or trademarked medication
   k. conforming to instructions; obedient; observant
   l. person—resistant to authority; illness—resistant to treatment; stubborn

Chapter 3

A. Multiple Choice
1. B
2. D
3. A

B. Short Answer
1. Diseases may be hereditary, familial, or environmental.
2. Age and health or age at death and cause of death of immediate family members are included.
3. A sibling is a brother or sister.
4. A hereditary disease is transmissible from parent to offspring by information encoded in the parents' genes.

Chapter 4

A. Multiple Choice
1. A
2. B

B. Short Answer
An ideal Social History includes data on the patient's birth, upbringing, academic career, marital history and present status, spouse's health history, military service, occupations past and present, avocations and hobbies, social and cultural pursuits, political and religious activities, foreign travel or residence, financial status, police record, and current family structure, living arrangements, and personal responsibilities.

Chapter 5

A. Multiple Choice
1. B
2. D

B. Fill in the Blank
1. lifestyle
2. caffeine
3. eating disorders
4. alcohol; drugs
5. pack-year
6. prescription; nonprescription

C. Short Answer
1. Types of medications include pills, capsules, liquids, ointments, eye or nose drops, inhalers, and patches. Oral contraceptives, vitamins, laxatives, and headache and cold remedies are often omitted. A satisfactory medication record includes the (generic) name of the drug, dosage form, strength, frequency of use, and the reason for which it was prescribed.
2. Clues include a history of drinking alone, drinking in the morning to get started or to stop shaking, blackouts or spells of amnesia, arrests for public drunkenness or drunk driving, and adverse effects of drinking on work, family and social relationships.
3. a. restraint; avoidance of
   b. eating disorder associated with life-threatening weight loss
   c. eating disorder often involving bingeing and then purging either by vomiting or abusing laxatives
   d. sleeplessness; wakefulness
   e. sleepwalking
   f. inactive
   g. verbose; wordy; talkative
   h. alcoholism
   i. packs per day times total years smoked

Chapter 6

A. Multiple Choice
1. C
2. E
3. D

B. Fill in the Blank
1. relevant
2. negatives
3. crucial; critical

C. Short Answer
1. Even the most minor surgical procedure may result in changes of structure or function that may later be mistaken for signs of disease.
2. a. consequence; result, especially pathological condition resulting from disease
   b. unusual individual reaction to food or drug
   c. cursory; superficial

Chapter 7

A. Multiple Choice
1. D
2. C
3. D
4. A
5. D

B. Fill in the Blank
1. systemic diseases
2. cardinal
3. brain tumor; diabetes
4. vertigo; dysequilibrium

C. Short Answer
1. warning
2. chief; principal; primary
3. zigzag banding of light marking the margins of the scintillating scotoma of migraine
4. an early or premonitory symptom of a disease
5. transient blindness
6. yellow vision
7. night blindness
8. sensation of spinning or whirling
9. acute rhinitis (inflammation of nasal membrane)
10. swallowing
11. dryness of the mouth
12. clenching or grinding the teeth

Chapter 8

A. Multiple Choice
1. A
2. C
3. D
4. B, D
5. A

B. Fill in the Blank
1. cardiovascular disorders
2. upright
3. pillows
4. structures
5. (intermittent) claudication
6. congestive heart failure

C. Short Answer
1. Categories include coronary arteriosclerosis, valvular heart disease, hypertension, congestive heart failure, pericardial disease, local or generalized arteriosclerosis, and venous disease.
2. Parameters are character, intensity, location, extent, radiation, duration, frequency; effect of position, movement, breathing, and swallowing; associated symptoms; the effect of resting or taking medicines; and triggering factors.
3. It is graded by how far or how many flights of stairs a patient can walk before experiencing symptoms.
4. The danger of pulmonary embolism with deep vein thrombosis makes every complaint of peripheral swelling significant.
5. a. discomfort on breathing when lying flat
   b. limping
   c. functional murmur, not associated with a heart lesion
   d. shortness of breath

Chapter 9

A. Multiple Choice
1. C
2. C

B. Fill in the Blank
1. tracheobronchial tract; lungs
2. asthma; bronchitis
3. expectorated (material)
4. pain-sensitive

C. Short Answer
1. lung condition causing wheezing
2. bronchial tube inflammation
3. coughing up blood

Chapter 10

A. Multiple Choice
1. D
2. C
3. A, B
4. C

B. Fill in the Blank
1. lips
2. food
3. flatulence
4. bile pigment

C. Short Answer
1. The two primary symptoms are abdominal pain and digestive system disturbance. Disorders of the liver or biliary tract, pancreas, rectum, or anus are also covered.
2. They mean different things to different people. The patient would be questioned about the frequency and consistency of stools.
3. a. blood in vomitus
   b. blood in stool
   c. excessive hunger
   d. craving/eating non-nutritive substances like chalk or paint
   e. growling sound in intestines
   f. hiccups

Chapter 11

A. Multiple Choice
1. E
2. C
3. D

B. Fill in the Blank
1. kidneys; urinary tract; reproductive system
2. reproductive
3. ureters; bladder; urethra
4. nocturia
5. menarche

C. Short Answer
1. A GU history includes past diagnoses of congenital anomalies of the urinary or genital tract; urinary tract infections; stone in a kidney, ureter, or bladder; sexually transmitted diseases; genitourinary surgery; and menstrual and reproductive history.
2. It includes flank pain, frequency, nocturia, pain, burning, difficulty voiding, diminution in stream, incontinence, bedwetting, blood in urine, or other change in appearance of urine.
3. It includes pregnancies, miscarriages, abortions, stillbirths, normal and cesarean births, and any complications of pregnancy.
4. Symptoms include contraceptive use; pelvic pain, vaginal discharge, vulvar itching, sores, or rash; and any breast complaints.
5. Symptoms include urethral discharge or burning; itching, rash, ulcers, nodules, or other lesions of the genitals; pain or swelling in the testicles; scrotal masses; and infertility.
6. a. urination
   b. birth defect
   c. urine stone
   d. unduly frequent urination
   e. urinary incontinence
   f. scant urine production
   g. no urine production
   h. menses
   i. menopause
   j. breast development
   k. masturbation

Chapter 12

A. Multiple Choice
1. A
2. D
3. B

B. Fill in the Blank
1. paresthesia
2. central; peripheral

C. Short Answer
1. They include severe or unusual headache; unexplained drowsiness or dysequilibrium; confusion; disorientation; sudden deterioration of memory, judgment, or emotional stability; tremors; incoordination; disorders of speech; weakness, clumsiness, paralysis, or spasticity of the extremities; and seizures.
2. a. ataxia; inability to coordinate muscle movements
   b. marked by intervals
   c. in the past
   d. lack of balance
   e. loss of consciousness
   f. to draw forth; bring out
   g. making less severe or less painful
   h. hooklike or hook-shaped
3. Symptoms include crying out, falling, loss of consciousness, confusion, twitching, writhing, incontinence, weakness, and drowsiness.

Chapter 13

A. Fill in the Blank
1. historian
2. psychiatrist
3. interview

B. Short Answer
1. Subjects include prior diagnosis of mental, emotional, or nervous illness and treatments used, including counseling, group therapy, drug therapy, hospitalization, and electroshock; family and marital harmony; school performance; job stability and satisfaction; social contacts; sleep pattern; drug and alcohol use; and general sense of well-being, self-esteem, and purpose in life.
2. A person with even a mild mood or personality disorder frequently resists talking about it, and a person with severe psychiatric impairment makes a most unreliable historian.
3. a. perception of an object or event that isn't really there
   b. extreme apprehension
   c. unfounded or irrational fear
   d. having two extremes, as in mania and depression
   e. chronic mood disorder
   f. false belief
   g. a type of psychosis
   h. progressive loss of cognitive and intellectual function
   i. psychological needs expressed with physical symptoms
   j. indifference; lack of interest

Chapter 14

A. Multiple Choice
1. C
2. B

B. Fill in the Blank
1. systemic
2. cutaneous; skin

C. Short Answer
1. They are local or general eruptions or rashes, itching, dryness or scaling, pigment changes, and solid tumors of various kinds.
2. The examiner will ask about prior diagnoses and any treatments used; the duration of the problem; whether it comes and goes, remains unchanged, or is gradually getting better or worse; whether it is spreading from one area to others; whether the patient can suggest any reason for the problem; and whether anything seems to make the problem better or worse.
3. a. relating to the skin
   b. inherited condition characterized by scaly lesions
   c. hypersensitive to environmental allergens
   d. rash; breaking out
   e. self-induced
   f. destruction of lesions by electric current
   g. viral skin eruption
   h. crust developing over a burn
   i. excess body hair, especially in women
   j. boil
   k. formation of pus
   l. mole
   m. scar

Chapter 15

A. Multiple Choice
1. C
2. D
3. A
4. C

B. Fill in the Blank
1. ballottement
2. fluctuancy
3. rebound
4. cyst
5. brachial
6. diastolic

C. Short Answer
1. a. instrument used to measure thickness
   b. a flat glass plate used to examine skin lesions under pressure
   c. measures blood pressure; an inflatable cuff, bulb, and gauge
   d. a device used to study the interior of the eye through the pupil
   e. underlying reason
   f. fateful; foreshadowing disaster
   g. fixed; unchanging
   h. wound; injury; pathologic change in tissue
   i. expressible in terms of quantity; measurable
   j. vibration
   k. irregular; unusual; deviated from normal
   l. acquiring masculine physical traits
   m. spindle-shaped
   n. swollen; congested; edematous
2. Regardless of the sequence in which data are obtained, they are generally recorded in a format that begins with the general appearance and skin and then progresses from the head and face to the extremities, followed by the neurologic and psychiatric categories. This follows a pattern of going from the outside to the inside and from top to bottom (head to toe).

Chapter 16

A. Multiple Choice
1. C
2. C

B. Fill in the Blank
1. psychiatric; mental status
2. mental state

C. Short Answer
1. General features include body build, nutritional status, apparent age, and general state of health, skin color, alertness and responsiveness, mood, posture, gait, mobility, grooming, and personal hygiene, quality and clarity of voice and speech, evidence of distress, abnormal orders of breath or body, and other readily observable abnormalities.
2. a. physical characteristic; body build
   b. thin; delicate body type
   c. endomorphic; rounded and ample
   d. with signs and symptoms of Cushing disease
   e. cachexic; suffering from marasmus
   f. weight loss and wasting
   g. mentally dulled
   h. obesity
   i. high-pitched noisy respiration
   j. containing or forming pus
   k. generalized edema of subcutaneous connective tissue
   l. sweating; perspiring
   m. stiff, short-stepped gait of parkinsonism

Chapter 17

A. Multiple Choice

1. D
2. A
3. B
4. A
5. C

B. Fill in the Blank

1. petechia
2. excoriation or abrasion

C. Short Answer

1. A first-degree burn is characterized by erythema (redness), a second-degree burn by blistering, and a third-degree burn by charring.
2. A keloid is thicker than a regular scar and can be painful.
3. a. skin
   b. freckle
   c. smooth; hairless
   d. horny skin lesion
   e. abnormal passage
   f. cell death; dead tissue
   g. calculus or stone
   h. fatty tumor
   i. large area of subcutaneous edema; allergic reaction
   j. fullness
   k. appearance of a tent when skin is picked up
   l. abnormal formation of fibrous tissue
   m. enlargement; increase in bulk
   n. redness of the skin
   o. blueness of the skin
   p. area of skin covered with macular lesions of varying shades and colors

Chapter 18

A. Multiple Choice

1. B
2. C
3. D

B. Fill in the Blank

1. congenital
2. malignancy
3. carotid

C. Short Answer

1. The face often reflects systemic disease in addition to the current emotional state.
2. Neck motion may be restricted due to joint stiffness, muscle spasm, or pain.
3. The neck supports the head, is the channel for nerve connections between brain and body, and supplies a passageway for the exchange of gases (oxygen and carbon dioxide), blood flow, and food and drink.
4. a. neck spasm
   b. back of the head
   c. relating to wall of a cavity or to parietal bone
   d. projecting point of the forehead
   e. shortness of the head
   f. rounded swelling
   g. baldness; loss of hair
   h. patches of loss of pigment in hair
   i. involuntary repetitive movement
   j. zygomatic bone; cheek bone
   k. wrinkled; shrunken
   l. wan; dull
   m. skull anomaly; basilar invagination
   n. inflammation and fissures at corners of the mouth
   o. chewing
   p. dry, waxy swelling of skin associated with hypothyroidism

Chapter 19

A. Multiple Choice

1. D
2. B
3. A
4. A

B. Fill in the Blank

1. scotomata
2. glaucoma
3. fluorescein
4. abnormal sensitivity
5. Snellen wall chart; Jaeger test types

C. Short Answer

1. a. nontransparent
   b. artificial body part
   c. meibomian cyst; tarsal cyst
   d. tearing
   e. rhythmic/jerky eye movements
   f. nearsightedness
   g. farsightedness
   h. corneal warping
   i. crossed eyes; heterotropia
   j. increased convexity of the lens
   k. loss of vision in half the visual field
   l. age-related visual deterioration; old eyes

Chapter 20

A. Multiple Choice

1. B
2. C
3. D
4. C

B. Fill in the Blank

1. cartilage
2. Rinne; Weber
3. otoscope

C. Short Answer

1. Conductive hearing loss results from disease or injury of middle ear structures; neurosensory loss results from malfunction of the acoustic nerve due to aging, noise exposure, or drug/chemical exposure.
2. external ear; middle ear; inner ear
3. Visible on exam are lack of mobility, injection, bulging, retraction, perforation, discoloration, fluid level, bubbles, tumors, scars, and a PE tube.
4. a. elevated cartilage opposite the helix
   b. the difference in hearing via air and bone conduction
   c. middle ear mass from chronic otitis media
   d. forced expiratory effort on a closed airway; straining
   e. test of hearing with an electrical instrument (audiometer)
   f. heel-to-toe walking
   g. manner of walking
   h. a state of balance
   i. unit for expressing loudness
   j. ear discharge

Compare and Contrast

The term "eardrum" (Greek *tympanon*) refers to the entire middle ear, which is somewhat stretched across its only open side. The tympanic membrane is not the drum, but only the drumhead or skin (to use terms that a percussionist might use). The tympanic membrane is the only part of the eardrum that can be seen on exam so this term is often used synonymously with "eardrum," although they are not the same.

Chapter 21

A. Multiple Choice

1. C
2. D
3. B

B. Fill in the Blank

1. mirror
2. buccal
3. skull

C. Short Answer

1. The physician looks for developmental abnormalities, traumatic deformities, enlargement, nodules, ulcers, and lesions.
2. A small light is placed against part of the head and face or inside the mouth in a dark room; a deep ruddy glow can be seen through the skin when the sinuses are filled with air. The intensity and configuration of the flow are different when the sinuses are filled with pus or mucus.
3. Contributing to bad breath are ketosis, uremia, hepatic failure, dental disease, oral disease, and infection in the respiratory tract.
4. a. white patch on the mucous membrane
   b. small nipple-like structure
   c. shedding; casting off
   d. inflammation of the tongue
   e. oropharyngeal passage
   f. fluid exuded from tissue
   g. containing or forming pus
   h. nasal openings

Chapter 22

A. Multiple Choice

1. A
2. B

B. Fill in the Blank

1. emphysema
2. neck; diaphragm

C. Short Answer

1. Visual inspection can show configuration of the chest walls and any deformity; breathing movements; skin lesions, scars, swellings or obvious tumors; pigment and hair distribution; and breast size and symmetry.
2. a. sword shaped; xiphoid process is cartilage at the end of the sternum
   b. collar bone
   c. relating to a rib
   d. suffering from rickets
   e. auxiliary
   f. involuntary rigidity of muscles to palpation
   g. stiffening of body part to avoid pain
   h. exceeding the normal number; extra
   i. one quarter of a circle; a division for descriptive purposes; 1/4
   j. armpits
   k. sagging; greatly relaxed

Chapter 23

A. Multiple Choice

1. A
2. A
3. D
4. C

B. Fill in the Blank

1. S1
2. systole
3. carotid
4. heart sounds

C. Short Answer

1. They are designated as mitral, pulmonic, aortic, and tricuspid.
2. Crescendo starts soft and grows louder; decrescendo starts loud and grows softer; crescendo-decrescendo becomes first louder, then softer.
3. a. slight sharp sound
   b. friction sound
   c. tip or summit
   d. seemingly contradictory
   e. pairing
   f. related only to the ventricles
   g. epigastric and anterior surface of the lower part of the thorax
   h. a gradual increase
   i. a triple cadence to the heart sounds

Chapter 24

A. Multiple Choice

1. C
2. C
3. A

B. Fill in the Blank

1. vesicular
2. (vocal) fremitus

C. Short Answer

1. Breathing through the mouth avoids extraneous sounds caused by the passage of air through the nose.
2. They include collapse of lung tissue or lung collapse (atelectasis); consolidation due to pneumonia; the presence of air (pneumothorax), blood (hemothorax), pus (empyema) or fluid (hydrothorax, pleural effusion) in the pleural space; and tumor.
3. a. from an external source
   b. bubbly noise; rale
   c. increased transmission of voice sound through pulmonary structures
   d. shaking to elicit a splashing sound
   e. broken quality to the voice; bleating
   f. increased intensity of voice heard over a bronchus
   g. vibration imparted to the hand
   h. incomplete lung expansion; lung collapse
   i. pleural fluid

Chapter 25

A. Multiple Choice

1. B
2. C
3. D
4. D

B. Fill in the Blank

1. bowel
2. lithotomy
3. rectocele
4. Leopold

C. Short Answer

1. Assessment is made of skin turgor and muscle tone; size, shape, and position of the abdominal and pelvic organs; any masses, pulsations, and tenderness.
2. They consist of the ovaries, tubes, broad ligaments, round ligaments, and associated blood vessels.
3. a. lying face up
   b. belly button
   c. dilated veins
   d. an opening
   e. boat-shaped; concave
   f. layer of tissue; apron
   g. gallbladder removal
   h. abnormal enlargement of an organ
   i. movement of the intestine; waves
   j. inflammation of the penis or clitoris
   k. undescended testicle(s)
   l. inflammation of the epididymis
   m. removal of a stone
   n. pubic hair
   o. lice infestation
   p. benign uterine tumor
   q. ringlike band of muscle fibers
   r. piles

Chapter 26

A. Multiple Choice
1. A
2. D
3. B

B. Fill in the Blank
1. passive
2. goniometer
3. edema

C. Short Answer
1. It is judged by its color.
2. Blood flow is determined in major arteries through palpation and grading of pulses and auscultation for bruits. Capillary circulation is assessed by compression and refill and the Allen test. Adson test is performed. Varicose veins, if present, are tested with Trendelenburg and Brodie tests.
3. a. pertaining to the back
   b. pertaining to the belly
   c. relating to the sole of the foot
   d. relating to the palm or sole
   e. relating to the palm of the hand
   f. nearest the point of origin
   g. away from the point of origin
   h. full of twists and turns
   i. thickening and widening of the digits
   j. relating to the feet
   k. movement of a body part away from the median plane
   l. movement of a body part toward the median plane
   m. movement of a part in a circular direction
   n. progressive enlargement of the head, hands, and feet
   o. emaciation; gradual loss of weight and strength
   p. wasting of tissue, organs, or the whole body

Chapter 27

A. Multiple Choice
1. D
2. D
3. B, D
4. C

B. Fill in the Blank
1. spinal cord
2. reflex
3. pathologic
4. resting

C. Short Answer
1. Assessed are size and reactivity of pupils, rate and rhythm of breathing, response to noxious stimuli (loud noise, firm pressure over bones), primitive reflexes (corneal and gag reflex), and doll's eye maneuver.
2. When the head is moved from side to side, the eyes rotate in a direction opposite the movement, maintaining the direction of gaze.
3. It provides information about muscle mass, strength, tone, and control.
4. a. waxing rigidity of the limbs
   b. progressive weakness and atrophy of the muscles of the tongue, lips, palate, pharynx, and larynx
   c. disorder of the spinal nerve roots
   d. difficulty in performing voluntary movements
   e. rigidity
   f. disorder of voluntary movement
   g. inability to coordinate muscle activity
   h. inflowing; denoting certain nerves
   i. walking so as to lessen pain
   j. relating to the cremaster muscle
   k. neurologic symptoms (e.g., positive Babinski) indicating a problem in the pyramidal tract of the brain
   l. reflex; scratching the palm results in contraction of some facial muscles
   m. inability to perform rapid alternating movements

n. disturbance of muscular coordination
o. sense of perception of movement
p. relating to the back of the neck
q. neurological syndrome characterized by severe spasms

Chapter 28

A. Multiple Choice
1. C
2. A
3. B

B. Fill in the Blank
1. mood
2. triad
3. memory

C. Short Answer
1. What is the time/day/month/year? Where are you? (city, state, exact present location) What is your name? What are the names of your family members and friends?
2. The format typically includes appearance, sensorium, activity and behavior, mood, thought content, intellectual function orientation, memory, judgment, and insight.
3. a. relating to touch
   b. inability to recognize sensory stimuli
   c. paralysis on one side of the body
   d. involuntary parroting of someone else's speech; echoing
   e. involuntarily performing motor or verbal acts
   f. relating to a disturbance of speech and language
   g. absence of pleasure
   h. formation of ideas or thoughts
   i. inability to perform simple mathematics
   j. a condition in children in which they are unresponsive to human contact
   k. compulsion to pull out one's own hair

Chapter 29

A. Multiple Choice

1. A
2. C

B. Fill in the Blank

1. milestones
2. head

C. Short Answer

1. Of concern are jaundice, respiratory distress, feeding difficulties, fever, and seizures.
2. These include the Moro (startle), grasp, rooting, and tonic neck reflexes.
3. a. membranous interval on skull; soft spot
   b. protuberance
   c. membrane fold supporting the tongue
   d. laryngotracheobronchitis
   e. baby's first bowel movement
   f. congenital herniation of internal organs
   g. webbing of fingers or toes
   h. congenital hypothyroidism
   i. paralysis of corresponding parts on both sides of the body
   j. pregnancy
   l. cat cry syndrome

Chapter 30

A. Multiple Choice

1. B
2. D
3. D

B. Fill in the Blank

1. diagnosis
2. prognosis

C. Short Answer

1. It means a diagnosis, although less than probable, remains a possibility for further consideration.
2. If they expect to be paid, they must speak the same diagnostic language as the prospective payer.
3. Numerical coding streamlines many aspects of health information management, including third-party payment, classification and analysis, peer review, and so on.
4. a. autopsy; after death
   b. a set system of names used in a science
   c. condition following as a consequence of a disease
   d. widely scattered
   e. between acute and chronic
   f. originating from within
   g. occurring suddenly and rapidly
   h. obstruction of a vessel by a clot
   i. a collection of four things having something in common
   j. faking illness to avoid work or gain sympathy
   k. changeable in form
   l. spread of disease from one part of the body to another

Index

About the Author

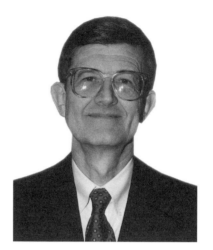

John H. Dirckx, M.D., has been director of the student health center at the University of Dayton in Dayton, Ohio, since 1968. His longstanding interest in classical and modern languages has led to the writing of several books and numerous articles on the language, literature, and history of medicine.

He is author of *The Language of Medicine: Its Evolution, Structure, and Dynamics*, 2nd ed. (New York: Praeger Publishers, 1983), *Roundsmanship: An Introductory Manual* (Modesto, Ca.: Health Professions Institute, 1987), *Laboratory Medicine: Essentials of Anatomic and Clinical Pathology*, 2nd ed. (Modesto, Ca.: Health Professions Institute, 1995), and *Human Diseases* (Modesto, Ca.: Health Professions Institute, 1997).

He is a frequent contributor of educational articles on medicine and medical language to medical transcription periodicals, including *Perspectives on the Medical Transcription Profession* (published by Health Professions Institute) and *Journal of AAMT* (American Association for Medical Transcription), and is medical consultant for *The SUM Program for Medical Transcription Training* developed by Health Professions Institute. He has also served as editor or consultant for several Stedman's publications. In addition, his short fiction appears regularly in national magazines.

His hobbies include book-collecting and music. He and his wife Joyce (to whom this book is dedicated) have five daughters and nine grandchildren.